Concepts of Addictive Substances and Behaviours across Time and Place

Governance of Addictive Substances and Behaviours Series

Series Editors: Peter Anderson and Antoni Gual

Titles in the series

Governance of Addictions: European Public Policies
Tamyko Ysa, Joan Colom, Adrià Albareda, Anna Ramon, Marina Carrión, and Lidia Segura

The Impact of Addictive Substances and Behaviours on Individual and Societal Well-being
Edited by Peter Anderson, Jürgen Rehm, and Robin Room

What Determines Harm from Addictive Substances and Behaviours?
Edited by Lucy Gell, Gerhard Bühringer, Jane McLeod, Sarah Forberger, John Holmes, Anne Lingford-Hughes, and Petra Meier

Concepts of Addictive Substances and Behaviours across Time and Place

Edited by

Matilda Hellman

Virginia Berridge

Karen Duke

Alex Mold

OXFORD
UNIVERSITY PRESS

OXFORD
UNIVERSITY PRESS

Great Clarendon Street, Oxford, OX2 6DP,
United Kingdom

Oxford University Press is a department of the University of Oxford.
It furthers the University's objective of excellence in research, scholarship,
and education by publishing worldwide. Oxford is a registered trade mark of
Oxford University Press in the UK and in certain other countries

First Edition published in 2016

Published in the United States of America by Oxford University Press
198 Madison Avenue, New York, NY 10016, United States of America

British Library Cataloguing in Publication Data
Data available

Library of Congress Control Number: 2015948867

ISBN 978-0-19-873779-7

Foreword

This book, *Concepts of Addictive Substances and Behaviours across Time and Place*, is the fourth in a series of six books arising out of ALICE RAP (Addictions and Lifestyles in Contemporary Europe—Reframing Addictions Project), a five-year, €10 million endeavour co-financed by the Social Sciences and Humanities division of FP7 within the European Commission, and led by the Clínic Foundation for Biomedical Research based in Barcelona and the Institute of Health and Society in Newcastle University (http://wwww.alicerap.eu). The first book described current European approaches to governing addictive substances and behaviours (Ysa et al., 2014). The second book described the impact of addictive substances and behaviours on individual and societal well-being (Anderson et al., 2015). The third book documented determinants of harm (Meier et al., 2015). The remaining two books will address the impact of market forces on addictive substances and behaviours, and a new governance of addictive substances and behaviours.

ALICE RAP studies the place of addictions and lifestyles in contemporary Europe and aims to inform how we can better redesign their governance. By addictions, we mean the regular and sustained heavy use of drugs, such as alcohol, nicotine, and cocaine, and regular and sustained heavy engagement in actions such as gambling or Internet gaming.

The use of psychoactive substances in Europe is linked to considerable harm, millions of years lived with disability, millions of years lost due to premature death, and social costs in the hundreds of billions of euros (Anderson et al., 2015). Harm affects all aspects of life; harm is due not just to the drugs themselves, but also to the way that societies deal with psychoactive substances. Harm results from a complex interplay between cellular and molecular determinants, individual determinants, and social and environmental determinants (Meier et al., 2015).

It is reasonable to say that no one European country yet has it right in their governance approach to addictions, although those that implement a well-being and relational management strategy embracing a comprehensive policy for addictions lead the way (Ysa et al., 2014). Such countries tend to be those in which the ministry of health, as opposed to the ministry of the interior, is the main body responsible for planning and implementing drug policy; have a harm reduction as opposed to a regulatory approach; decriminalize as opposed to criminalize drug use; have proactive as opposed to reactive policymaking;

have a health-oriented rather than public-security approach; and aim to protect the public and society in general rather than focus on individual responsibility. Countries which embrace a comprehensive policy for addictions tend to tackle licit and illicit substances together, as opposed to split substance policies; have a long experience in drug and addiction policies, as opposed to little experience and poor continuity; have a complexity rather than simplicity in organizational structures; have multilevel governance and high levels of devolution, rather than centralized organizational structures; and involve rather than exclude stakeholders. Since only just over one-quarter of the twenty-eight European countries studied fall in the well-being and relational management strategy/comprehensive policy for addictions cluster, there is clearly an enormous opportunity for improvement for Europe as a whole (Ysa et al., 2014).

However, if we are ever to improve our governance of addictions, we need to understand the starting points, reflected in the mosaic of Europe. How does the 'ownership of addiction' vary across time and place? In a unique and readable way, this book does just that, by analyzing concepts in both national and global policies (e.g. Hellman et al., 2016; Taylor et al., 2016), and by tying these concepts to certain stakeholders (e.g. Bjerge et al., 2016; Houborg et al., 2016), professional groups (e.g. Egerer et al., 2016), and cultural contexts (e.g. Blomqvist et al., 2016). On the one hand, the book points out an enormous mosaic: with understandings of what addiction is varying dramatically over time and place; with the importance of different stakeholder groups waxing and waning over time and place; with images of addiction varying enormously across professional and lay groups, often at variance with the harm done by different substances and behaviours. On the other hand, it points out that the ownership of addiction is driven by forces that diminish variation in the mosaic: by the English language, by the biological sciences, and by 'global epistemic governance', by which is meant governance that works by

> influencing other actors' beliefs and views of the way in which the social world is organized, the role and subject positions of actors, and the nature of ethical or valued goals of social change. In other words, epistemic work revolves around constructions of what the world is, who we are, and what is good or desirable. (Alasuutari & Qadir, 2014, p. 78)

I would argue that we need both approaches. On the one hand, a mosaic opens up opportunities for all sorts of natural experiments for analyzing the impact of different approaches in reducing harm (Anderson & Room, 2011), provided, of course, that parts of the mosaic do no harm—which is, unfortunately, not the case. There are too many examples of addiction policies that stigmatize and criminalize users of drugs, and fail to provide evidence-based help and treatment for those who would benefit, leading to many lost years of poor health and well-being (Moskalewicz & Klingemann, 2015; Stoll & Anderson, 2015).

On the other hand, biological understanding of addictions can drive public good. Evolutionary biology's findings that we humans have evolved to counter-exploit potent plant neurotoxins—including nicotine, morphine, and cocaine—to our advantage, suggests that we are active and functional in relation to the drugs that we take, rather than passive and vulnerable (Sullivan & Hagen, 2015). This would suggest, as the evidence demonstrates, that prohibition is likely to fail, because substance use is not 'caused' by biological frailty in people in general. Toxicological analysis is a method for estimating the potency of the different drugs we take by comparing the ratio of their toxic dose with the dose consumed (Lachenmeier & Rehm, 2015). Such analyses tend to show dissonances between drug potency on the one hand and the potency of policy responses on the other. That we are social animals confirms the power of our social networks in impacting our individual behaviours (Christakis & Fowler, 2008; Rosenquist et al., 2010).

If we are going to move forward for a better governance of addictions, we need a unifying concept that works across time and place, and works across the molecular, individual, and social determinants of harm. Elsewhere, we have argued that 'heavy use over time' is that unifying concept (Rehm et al., 2013; Rehm et al., 2014). Heavy use over time is consistent with recent advancements in biological sciences; it fits better into the approach of public health, being more closely linked to health and social consequences; it is clinically applicable in health systems, with easy operationalization and with sufficient interventions; and it promises to reduce stigmatization, as it is based on a truly continuous variable.

However, if we are going to be able to map convergence of the concept of heavy use over time across time and place, we need to understand the existing mosaic—this book helps us do just that.

Peter Anderson
International Coordinator of the ALICE RAP project; Chief Series Editor, Governance of Addictive Substances and Behaviours; Professor, Substance Use, Policy, and Practice, Newcastle University, England; Professor, Alcohol, and Health, Maastricht University, Netherlands.

References

Alasuutari, P., & Qadir, A. (2014). Epistemic governance: an approach to the politics of policy-making. *European Journal of Cultural and Political Sociology*, **1**(1), 67–84.

Anderson, P., Rehm, J., & Room, R. (Eds.). (2015). *The impact of addictive substances and behaviours on individual and societal well-being.* Oxford, UK: Oxford University Press.

Anderson, P., & Room, R. (2011). Addictions and European policy: has the 'European project' stifled science-led policy? *Drug and Alcohol Review*, **30**, 117–118.

Bjerge, B., Duke, K., Asmussen Frank, V., Rolando, S. & Eisenbach-Stangl, I. (2016). Exploring user groups as stakeholders in drug policy processes in four European countries. In M. Hellman et al (Eds), *Concepts of addictive substances and behaviours across time and place*. Oxford: Oxford University Press. 107–128.

Blomqvist, J., Raitasalo, K., Melberg, H.O., Schreckenberg, D., Peschel, C., Klingemann, J., et al. (2016). Popular images of addiction in five European countries. In M. Hellman et al. (Eds.), *Concepts of addictive substances and behaviours across time and place*. Oxford: Oxford University Press. 193–211.

Christakis, N.A., & Fowler, J.H. (2008). The collective dynamics of smoking in a large social network. *New England Journal of Medicine*, **358**, 2249–2258.

Egerer, M., Hellman, M., Bujalski, M., & Rolando, S. (2016). General practitioners' position on problematic gambling in three European welfare states. In M. Hellman et al. (Eds.), *Concepts of addictive substances and behaviours across time and place*. Oxford: Oxford University Press. 169–192.

Hellman, M., Hakkarainen, P., & Sæbø, G. (2016). Underpinnings of tobacco policy: an epistemic governance perspective. In M. Hellman et al. (Eds.), *Concepts of addictive substances and behaviours across time and place*. Oxford: Oxford University Press. 151–167.

Houborg, E., Thom, B., Beccaria, F. Eisenbach-Stangl, I., Herring, R., Moskalewicz, M., et al. (2016). The role of stakeholders in addictions policy and intervention. In M. Hellman et al. (Eds.), *Concepts of addictive substances and behaviours across time and place*. Oxford: Oxford University Press. 87–106.

Lachenmeier, D.W., & Rehm, J. (2015). Comparative risk assessment of alcohol, tobacco, cannabis and other illicit drugs using the margin of exposure approach. *Scientific Reports*, **5**, 8126. doi:10.1038/srep08126

Meier, P.S., Bühringer, G., Gell, L., McLeod, J., Forberger, S., Holmes, J., et al. (2015). *What determines harm from addictive substances and behaviours?* Oxford, UK: Oxford University Press.

Moskalewicz, J., & Klingemann, J. (2015). Addictive substances and behaviours and social justice. In P. Anderson et al. (Eds.), *The impact of addictive substances and behaviours on individual and societal well-being*. Oxford, UK: Oxford University Press. 143–160.

Rehm, J., Anderson, P., Gual, A., Kraus, L., Marmet, S., Room, R., et al. (2014). The tangible common denominator of substance use disorders: a reply to commentaries to Rehm et al. (2013). *Alcohol and Alcoholism*, **49**, 118–122.

Rehm, J., Marmet, S., Anderson, P., Gual, A., Kraus, L., Nutt, D. J., et al. (2013). Defining substance use disorders: do we really need more than heavy use? *Alcohol and Alcoholism*, **48**, 633–640.

Rosenquist, J. N., Murabito, J., Fowler, J. H., & Christakis, N. A. (2010). The spread of alcohol consumption behaviour in a large social network. *Annals of Internal Medicine*, **152**, 426–433.

Stoll, L., & Anderson, P. (2015). Well-being as a frame for understanding addictive substances. In P. Anderson et al. (Eds.), *The impact of addictive substances and behaviours on individual and societal well-being*. Oxford, UK: Oxford University Press. 53–76.

Sullivan, R.J., & Hagen, E.H. (2015). Passive vulnerability or active agency? An ecological and evolutionary perspective on human drug use. In P. Anderson et al. (Eds.), *The impact of addictive substances and behaviours on individual and societal well-being*. Oxford, UK: Oxford University Press. 13–36.

Taylor, S., Berridge, V., & Mold, A. (2016). WHO expert committees and key concepts for drugs, alcohol, and tobacco, 1949–2013. In M. Hellman et al. (Eds.), *Concepts of addictive substances and behaviours across time and place*. Oxford: Oxford University Press. 57–85.

Ysa, T., Colom, J. Albareda, A., Ramon, A., Carrión, M., & Segura, L. (2014). *Governance of addictions: European public policies*. Oxford: Oxford University Press.

Acknowledgements

This research would not have been possible without financial support from the European Union, which funded the ALICE RAP project through the Seventh Framework Programme (FP7/2007–2013) under Grant Agreement 266813 (http://www.alicerap.eu). We would like to thank all colleagues in Area 1, ALICE RAP participants and colleagues at home institutions who have contributed to the development of our ideas through formal and informal discussions over the years.

Disclaimer

Contents

List of Contributors

Vibeke Asmussen Frank
Centre for Alcohol and Drug Research,
Aarhus University,
Denmark

Franca Beccaria
Eclectica, Institute for Training and Research,
Turin, Italy

Virginia Berridge
Centre for History in Public Health,
London School of Hygiene and Tropical Medicine,
UK

Bagga Bjerge
Centre for Alcohol and Drug Research,
Aarhus University,
Denmark

Jan Blomqvist
Centre for Social Research on Alcohol and Drugs, SoRAD,
Stockholm University,
Sweden

Michał Bujalski
Institute of Psychiatry and Neurology,
Warsaw, Poland

Karen Duke
Drug and Alcohol Research Centre, Middlesex University,
London, UK

Johan Edman
Centre for Social Research on Alcohol and Drugs, SoRAD,
Stockholm University,
Sweden

Michael Egerer
Department of Social Research,
University of Helsinki,
Finland

Irmgard Eisenbach-Stangl
European Centre for Social Welfare Policy and Research,
Vienna, Austria

Pekka Hakkarainen
National Institute for Welfare and Health, Helsinki,
Finland

Matilda Hellman
Department of Social Research,
University of Helsinki,
Finland

Grazyna Herczyńska
Institute of Psychiatry and Neurology,
Warsaw, Poland

Rachel Herring
Drug and Alcohol Research Centre,
Middlesex University,
London, UK

Esben Houborg
Centre for Alcohol and Drug Research, Aarhus University,
Denmark

Justyna Klingemann
Institute of Psychiatry and Neurology,
Warsaw, Poland

Anja Koski-Jännes
University of Tampere, Finland

Hans Olav Melberg
Department of Health Management and Health Economics,
University of Oslo,
Norway

Alex Mold
Centre for History in Public Health, London School of Hygiene and Tropical Medicine, UK

Jacek Moskalewicz
Institute of Psychiatry and Neurology,
Warsaw, Poland

Riikka Perälä
Department of Social Research, University of Helsinki, Finland

Christine Peschel
Zeus GmbH, Center for Applied Psychology, Environmental and Social Research, Hagen, Germany

Enrico Petrilli
Eclectica, Institute for Training and Research,
Turin, Italy

Kirsimarja Raitasalo
National Institute for Welfare and Health, Helsinki, Finland

Sara Rolando
Eclectica, Institute for Training and Research,
Turin, Italy

Gunnar Sæbø
State Institute for Drug Abuse (SIRUS),
Olso, Norway

Dirk Schreckenberg
Zeus GmbH, Center for Applied Psychology, Environmental and Social Research,
Hagen, Germany

Suzanne Taylor
London School of Hygiene and Tropical Medicine,
UK

Betsy Thom
Drug and Alcohol Research Centre, Middlesex University,
London, UK

Marta Welbel
Institute of Psychiatry and Neurology, Warsaw, Poland

Chapter 1

Ownership of addiction: variations across time and place

Matilda Hellman, Virginia Berridge, Karen Duke, and Alex Mold

1.1 A European perspective

This book focuses on historical and social scientific inquiries into the phenomenon of addiction in Europe. How the concept of addiction and addiction-related problems are viewed and addressed is never static; they vary over time and between cultures and countries. This statement may sound self-evident. But even a quick scan of the results generated by an Internet search brings the realization that the ownership of addiction research is mainly in the hands of forces that strive to discount variations. Mainstreaming forces of global epistemic governance, hard science research, and the English language dominate the doctrines of addiction research. Primary ownership of the addiction question is currently located in the influential 'evidence-based' policy movement geared to a problem-solving mode. The evidence-based paradigm, with origins in public health epidemiology, medicine, and psychology, has been tremendously important in raising political awareness and conceptualizing substance use, smoking, and gambling in a way that is adaptable to politics and praxis. As such, it has had great influence over the reduction of harm caused by addictive substances and behaviours. This circumstance will also be illustrated in many of the analyses contained within this volume. At the same time, the search for policy relevant and globally applicable knowledge may have pushed knowledge on cultural and social variations to the background. Complexity may have been lost in subtle but crucial dimensions.

The research in this volume is part of Area 1, 'Ownership of addiction', in a large-scale European seventh framework research project called Addictions and Lifestyles in Contemporary Europe—Reframing Addictions Project (ALICE RAP). The scholars of Area 1 in the ALICE RAP project recognized a great need to identify and emphasize the nuances that are often missing from the governing research on how addictions are viewed and addressed in Europe.

This is important not least because Europe is a continent with a variety of languages and cultures. During the five-year period 2011–2016, we have concentrated on three main areas.

First, we have studied the concepts of addiction over time and in different countries. Our research here has focused at the national country level; at the regional level; and internationally, through the lens of the key international organization, the World Health Organization (WHO). Here we have shown that the standard Anglo-American view of the developments of concepts of addiction from the mid-nineteenth century did not apply to all European countries. Different countries developed different concepts at different times, often arising out of local cultural traditions. Even the regional Nordic bloc, often spoken of as an entity, showed disparity over concepts related to drugs. The WHO played a universalizing role so far as concepts were concerned in the period after World War II. Greater homogeneity was achieved within Europe, but even so local traditions and the focus of policies remained different as late as the last decades of the twentieth century. We should accommodate and recognize these differences.

The second area of research is the governance of addiction, specifically focusing on the role and influence of different stakeholders in the development of policy and practice. Employing predominantly historical, policy science, and social science perspectives and qualitative case study designs, the research explored the role of stakeholders in opioid substitution treatment policy in Italy (Beccaria & Rolando, 2013), Denmark (Frank et al., 2013), the UK (Duke et al., 2013), Poland (Moskalewicz & Welbel, 2013) and Austria (Eisenbach-Stangl, 2013); in the Alcohol Health Alliance in the UK (Thom et al., in press, 2016); in drug consumption rooms in Denmark (Houborg & Frank, 2014; Houborg et al., 2014); in Italian alcohol policies (Beccaria & Rolando, 2014); in Austrian alcohol policy in the 1950s (Eisenbach-Stangl, forthcoming), in Polish alcohol policy in the 1980s (Moskalewicz & Welbel, 2014), and in heroin-assisted treatment at the supranational level (Duke, forthcoming). Different stakeholder groups were relevant in different contexts, in different countries, and at different periods in time. The research has illuminated the complex nature of policy making in this field and has deepened our understanding of stakeholder dynamics through an examination of the techniques by which particular groups try to gain power, build consensus, and shift the direction of policy. Often, their activities are facilitated by taking advantage of 'policy windows' or windows of opportunity opened by general political or ideological shifts to revise existing drug and alcohol strategies. Alliances or coalitions of stakeholders have also formed to advocate specific policy positions and build consensus over time. The ways in which the different stakeholder groups have produced, used, and disseminated evidence have been an important theme in our work (Duke & Thom, 2014; Thom et al., 2013). Our analyses have illustrated how particular forms of evidence and expertise are seen as more credible and legitimate than others in the development of policy. Some stakeholders, such as user groups, have struggled to be represented in the public debates and policy processes. On the other hand, there are also 'invisible' external stakeholder communities—the international organizations/agencies and donor countries—which have been powerful influences on internal national policies.

Governance of addiction and the concepts employed when speaking of the phenomenon cannot be separated from understandings of the behaviours. The third area of research in ALICE RAP Area 1 has thus been concerned with perceptions of addictions in different European countries—through the study of mass media portrayals (Beccaria et al., 2015; Bujalski et al., 2015; Hellman et al., 2015; Hellman & Room, 2014; Hellman 2013), of professionals' understandings of the problems (Hellman, 2015; Hellman et al., 2014; Egerer & Alanko 2015), and among general populations (Blomqvist et al., 2014). Many of the inquiries have their roots in the 'images theories of addiction' by Sulkunen (2015) which, during the past decade, has developed as a response to the essential challenges that have been brought against the addiction concept in social scientific inquiry. This conceptual approach does not require that addiction be a unitary condition to be real; addiction refers to a variety of phenomena, and is approached differently depending on the governing constructs that are applied (Sulkunen, 2015, p. 5). Nevertheless, the images research tradition (e.g. as developed in the Theories of Addiction and Images of Addictive Behaviours (IMAGES) consortium, 2007–2011; http://blogs.helsinki.fi/imagesofaddiction/) has not taken on a social constructionist approach in its most relativist sense. Instead, systematic analyses and mappings of cultural content, as well as professional and institutional views on the questions from different countries, have contributed to a greater understanding of rationales underpinning the variations and similarities of so-called addiction images (ideas, perceptions, understandings).

The three work packages accounted for in the preceding paragraphs underpin the structure of this book: the first part of the book consists of historical inquiries, the second focuses on stakeholders, and the third consists of inquiries from the images perspective. Each section and chapter can be read separately or as part of the larger entities.

1.2 **Concepts over time and place**

The concepts used to characterize 'addiction' are not value-free; nor are they static. The first section of the book (Chapters 2, 3, and 4) shows how these governing ideas change over time and place. We identify different types of location or state formation in which conceptual changes take place: Chapter 2 looks at the national level and at cross-national comparisons; Chapter 3 takes Nordic countries as a regional case study; and Chapter 4 looks at the role of an international body, the World Health Organization (WHO), in the period 1949–2013—at its international role in disseminating and consolidating common concepts which filtered down to the national level. These historical chapters examine drugs, alcohol, and tobacco, and identify similarities and divergences across the substances.

Our time frame in Chapter 2 begins in the mid-nineteenth century, when ideas about substance use as a disease first started to coalesce, and ends in the 1980s, when many countries across Europe were experiencing extended drug problems alongside traditional patterns of alcohol consumption. The chapter identifies three key periods when concepts changed: the 1860s to the 1920s and 30s, when ideas about disease and addiction were developing in North America and in Europe; the 1950s and 60s, the post–World War II years, when distinct national differences were still identifiable; and the 1970s and 80s, when greater uniformity and the influence of an international set of definitions was more visible, and when tobacco started to come onto the agenda. Our countries in this section are Austria, Italy, Poland, and the UK, providing a good cross-section of cultures, political systems, and patterns of substance use.

Our methods were unusual for historical work in that we aimed to use a common approach as far as possible, making use of the same types of source materials: medical journals and texts for the early period; policy documents and regulations for the later ones. The divergence across countries in both the availability and type of these sources was unexpected and a portent of the variance that started to emerge, once we looked at what the sources told us.

In the first period, the concept of 'inebriety' has dominated historical discussion and writing. But we found that this was a concept with an Anglo-American bias, which did not apply and was not so widely used in many European countries. Inebriety as an idea was located in the desire to do something about intemperance: a policy agenda to set up inebriate asylums which would treat alcohol abusers rather than imprison them. It had a strong moral and temperance focus within the medical framework. In European countries other than the UK, there were different influences. In Austria, for example, there was a domestic language surrounding 'drunkenness' as well as a more international terminology involving the notion of 'alcoholism'. There was also a parallel conceptual tradition in many countries, deriving from theories of insanity where the European influence was strong. 'Dipsomania' had a different heritage to inebriety. To this discussion of alcoholic insanity were added theories about hypodermic drug use; in particular, morphine. Discussion of 'morphinism' and 'morphinomania' partly originated in Germany and spread across Europe. So it was German scientific influence, rather than American or British, which held sway in much of continental Europe during the 1870s and 80s.

What was notable, too, was the role which different groupings and networks played in supporting and promoting different concepts. In the UK it was temperance-leaning doctors, from public health, general practice, or asylums. In Italy it was forensic scientists and theorists of degeneration (Beccaria & Petrilli, 2014; Berridge & Mold, 2014; Berridge et al., 2014; Eisenbach-Stangl, 2014; Moskalewicz & Herczyńska, 2014). Divergences were still present in policy documents from the 1950s and 60s. Alcohol was prominent as an issue in Poland, while drugs were central in occupied Austria, possibly because of U.S. influence. The British focus on tobacco, with the Royal College of Physicians' report in 1962, was not followed in the rest of Europe (Berridge, Mold, et al., 2014).

During the 1970s and 80s, differences between national contexts and across the substances remained. In Austria, drugs continued to attract more legislative attention than alcohol, whereas the opposite was true for Poland. Illicit drugs were also of significant interest in Italy, but primarily in connection with the international drug trade rather than domestic concerns about addiction. In Britain, alcohol and drugs were important policy issues, but so too was tobacco, a situation not found in the other European countries. A plethora of terms continued to exist to describe the problems connected to psychoactive substance use, but some degree of homogeneity could be found by the 1980s, as countries began to develop a common terminology under the influence of bodies such as the WHO and the European Monitoring Centre for Drugs and Drug Addiction (EMCDDA).

Chapter 3 looks at a regional bloc, the Nordic countries of Denmark, Sweden, and Finland. These countries are often identified as a regional entity, but analysis of the history of concepts and of policy for drugs shows divergences over time, but also a trend of policy convergence more recently. Again, theories of disease and addiction in the nineteenth century owed little to the Anglo-American tradition of inebriety. The language of 'morphinism' and 'morphinomania' was once more stimulated by German scientific thought. 'Narcomania' was a concept employed well into the twentieth century, and the term 'euphomania' was also put forward because of the use of different drugs, the amphetamines. But medical influence died away after World War II, when a more social approach in policy was established. Sweden and Finland operated in this period with a collective approach in policymaking, while Denmark focused on the needs of the individual. In more recent times, there is, however, a trend of greater similarity in policy across the three countries, although distinctive approaches have still been maintained. But this case study shows that there were commonalities across the Nordic countries and with the other case study countries in Europe, as well as distinct differences. We cannot easily speak of a regional response or conceptualization.

In Chapter 4 we examine the role of the WHO and its expert committees in the post–World War II period and the part these have played in establishing a more commonly accepted set of international definitions. This chapter shows that the language around drugs and the language around alcohol, although initially operating separately, both differentiated between 'addiction' and 'habit'. In the 1970s, attempts were made to develop a 'combined approach' to concepts and treatment. The concept of 'dependence'—discussed initially for drugs in the 1960s, later for alcohol—provided a unifying focus, which also began to be applied to tobacco. Tobacco had largely fallen outside these discussions and was rarely considered in European countries. Even in the initial UK policy document in 1962, 'habit' was the focus. Later there were attempts to apply 'dependence' to tobacco, which would have brought all three sets of substances—drugs, alcohol, and tobacco—together. But tobacco operated within a different framework: that of public health. Ideas about addiction arrived later and the policy route through the Framework Convention on Tobacco Control (FCTC) was different. The professionals who promoted the concepts were different, too, also at the national level —pharmacologists and psychiatrists on some of the drug and alcohol committees and public health professionals for tobacco.

The national chapters show that the influence of the WHO was growing throughout the post-war years and there was increasing homogeneity between countries. But the complexity of both national and international discussion over time, the change and variation in the networks which supported different concepts, and the rise and fall of conceptual frameworks, all demonstrate that time and place are crucial components of any discussion of addiction.

1.3 Governance and the role of stakeholders

The second part of the book focuses on the role of stakeholders in the development of policy and practice in the addictions fields. In Chapter 5, Houborg and his colleagues explore various conceptualizations of stakeholding by examining the different types of stakeholders in drug and alcohol policy, including institutions, professionals, experts, civic society, and corporations. The authors put forward a broad definition of stakeholders and distinguish between actors who can affect a policy and those who are affected by a policy issue. This distinction helps to highlight the issues of variable power and its distribution among stakeholder groups. They argue that the number of stakeholders in the addiction fields has increased dramatically as more and more behaviours, such as excessive gaming, Internet use, sex, shopping etc., have been problematized as 'addictions'. The increase in stakeholders is also linked to growing emphasis on democratic governance approaches that promote participation and the devolvement of power to municipal and local levels. This widens the stakeholder groups who have some opportunity to become engaged in governance at various levels. Drawing on case studies of stakeholders involved in opioid substitution treatment in Poland, Italy, Denmark, the UK, and Finland, the authors explore how stakeholder positions, legitimacy, and power are affected by wider political, social, and economic contexts. Also discussed are the ways stakeholders can use 'policy windows' to shift policy according to their ideological positions. These forms of stakeholder analyses highlight the context and conditions within which some stakeholder groups gain legitimacy and power to affect policy, while others are excluded from policy processes.

In Chapter 6, Bjerge and her colleagues conduct cross-national analyses of one stakeholder group—drug users in the UK, Denmark, Italy, and Austria. They illustrate how a relatively new category of stakeholders enters policy processes that traditionally have been occupied by politicians, social workers, legal actors, and/or medical doctors, and how the voices of citizens who are most affected by the laws and policies in the drug field can be included in the policy-making process. The authors explore how and why the levels of user participation, representation, and involvement in democratization processes vary from country to country. The analysis reveals that the four countries have very different traditions for involving users as stakeholders in policy processes. Although user groups influence the public debate and policy development in some countries, inclusion and influence in policy-making apparatuses is still variable and at a relatively low level: three of the countries are only beginning to grapple with the issues of representation, participation, and democratization, and one has not begun to do so.

In Chapter 7, Beccaria and her colleagues explore the impact of different kinds of external influences on internal national drug policy in Italy, Poland, Denmark, and Austria. They categorize these external influences into two groups: external *frameworks*, which include EU directives, strategies, WHO policy programmes, and UN Conventions, and external *stakeholders*, which include foreign governments, international agencies, and non-governmental organizations. The authors combine a number of theoretical perspectives to examine the role of external influences in national drugs policy governance. The four countries studied represent various welfare traditions and different drug epidemiology. The analysis indicates that national drug policies are strongly dependent on external influences, including UN agencies and individual countries such as the United States, which recommend different priorities in drug policy. At the same time, the 'authority' of external stakeholders can be employed in different ways by domestic stakeholders—to resist policy change and reinforce existing policy, or to legitimize a desired policy shift and use as a force to secure compliance.

1.4 **Images**

The third part of the book is concerned with conceptualizations per se, and specifically those that work as justifications in politics and governance, among welfare professionals, and among lay people in Europe today. Beccaria and colleagues already slightly opened the door, in Chapter 7, to the concept of *epistemic governance*. This is a recent sociological concept employed in neoinstitutional inquiries on how global forces of beliefs and knowledge 'work' perceptions of questions on different levels of policy making.

In Chapter 8, Hellman and her colleagues take on a clear case in which global epistemic governance has come to mark national strategies; namely, the tobacco control field. The authors inquire into tobacco policy justifications and discourses in Finland and Norway since the 1950s. They identify three stages of shifting focus regarding what the problem is about (*ontology*), who is affected and involved in solving it (*actor identification*), and the *normative aims* that these two stages suggest. The analysis shows the great rapidness with which tobacco policy was implemented, starting in the 1970s, with the aims of reducing harm for the smoker. Since World War II, public health research had found growing evidence of correlations between smoking and a series of diseases. Initially, reducing the harms caused by smoking was to be achieved primarily by targeting the individual smoker. In the second stage of tobacco control, a new aim was declared: a smoke-free society. In a radically new way, the concept of passive smoking strengthened demands for tighter tobacco regulations in many countries, so much so that in the second big wave of Finnish and Norwegian law reforms, in the mid-1990s, protection against the harms of passive smoking had become a central issue. The last stage of tobacco control has developed in a biological age, affirming individualized self-governance techniques and governing through body and brain (Hellman, 2013). Both harm reduction and a smoke-free society are strived for in tobacco policies, but in stage three tobacco control, Finland and Norway have focused on nicotine as an addictive substance that can overrule good intentions to stop smoking. Nicotine substitution therapy gained serious traction in the 1990s and has since permeated much of the way in which the tobacco problem is conceived. In the 2010s, the e-cigarette is not only a substitute for nicotine ingestion, it also replicates the oral sucking sensation and hand movements of the smoker, the authors observe. By discerning the logic underpinning tobacco policies, the chapter exposes the zeitgeist embedded in etiologies of the different eras.

Different images embedded in governance are also much in evidence in Chapter 9, where Egerer and his colleagues describe the nonstatic, culture-bound nature of ideas of gambling in the discourse of general practitioners (GPs). The authors describe focus group interviews with GPs from three countries—Finland, Italy, and Poland—during which interviewees were encouraged to talk freely about film clips depicting problematic gambling. The institutional context seemed to colour the views on the problems expressed by the professionals: Finnish GPs tended to replicate the Nordic welfare state's inclusive all-embracing system logic as well as some typical individual traits in that culture. The context of the Southern European welfare state was articulated in the Italian GPs' discourse about familial relations; the church was also seen to shape understandings of addiction. The Polish physicians referred to individual and familial contexts of help provision; as the authors explain, profound changes in Polish society have initiated changes in the perception of social problems, including their individualization. The findings of Chapter 9 strengthen the overall argument of the book by showing that cultural frameworks shape and permeate how addictive behaviours are understood (cf. Hellman & Room, 2014). It also points towards a conceptual influence by institutional practices on how problems are perceived (and vice versa). This circumstance will inevitably impose some challenges for any attempt to standardize the medical profession in addiction-related matters.

In the last chapter of the volume, Chapter 10, Blomqvist and his colleagues report on a survey that inquired into popular representations of addiction problems in five countries: Poland, Norway, Germany, Finland, and Sweden. The analyses indicate that there are large differences in the perceived severity of different addictions, and in the perceived addictiveness of various substances or activities. Addiction to 'hard' narcotic drugs (heroin, amphetamine, and cocaine) is, with few exceptions, seen as the most dangerous problem to society, whereas behavioural addictions, such as addictions to gambling and Internet use, generally come out as much less severe. Largely the same differences, although less pronounced, appear as concerns about the perceived risk of becoming addicted to various substances and/or activities. With respect to options for recovery, the confidence in treatment is relatively high for all addictions, whereas the chances for 'self-change' from addictions to 'hard' drugs—and to some extent medical drugs and alcohol—are generally rated as very or fairly small. On the other hand, the options of recovering from addictions to cigarettes or Internet use without treatment are generally rated as relatively high. Finally, most respondents seem to adopt a rather 'moral' view of addiction problems, holding the individual responsible both for acquiring and solving an addiction problem. The main exceptions here seem to be addictions to medical drugs, 'hard' narcotic drugs, and alcohol, where the individual is more often seen as a victim, and entitled to external help.

1.5 **Conclusions**

Based on the inquiries of this volume, it is clear that there are some interesting variances over time and space throughout Europe when it comes to understanding and addressing addiction problems. The reader may now well ask: what do all these variations in time and space mean and imply—for research, policy, and practice?

First, it tells us that addiction is neither a value-free concept nor as a phenomenon possible to be separated from its context. It is therefore unlikely that the multifaceted phenomenon of addiction can be fully understood and grasped through static (existing and future) models, especially if these lack complementary and explanatory knowledge of varying conceptions over time and space. If, for example, there were a global initiative to implement brief interventions for general practitioners (GPs) with respect to gambling problems, Chapter 9 shows that GPs in different countries will have different points of departure, elbow room, and scope for doing so. One can disregard heterogeneity and dynamics to a certain point, but in the long view, as long as the problems are socially, cognitively, and culturally articulated and construed, there will be an inevitable need to study and explain meaning-based variations in order to successfully address the problems.

As a follow-up to the necessity of studying the variations over time and place, we see that the variances imply the importance of the human and social sciences in the field of addiction studies. If we are to know and name the cultural and social dimensions, we need to give room to inquiries that are able to systematically map and explain them in accordance with standards in the fields of social sciences and humanities.

One implication of the actual variations across time and place is, of course, the changing landscape itself. We have shown that the stakeholders who are influential at the moment might not be so tomorrow. Change over time is central to historical understanding; we need to understand that concepts and the actors who promote them may themselves be time-limited. In the UK, the apparent decline of psychiatry as a lead discipline in addiction is one recent example.

In the studies presented in this book, the researchers have not asked, 'What is efficient?' or 'What is right?'; nor have they conducted randomized controlled trials for producing evidence of different techniques. Instead they have posed questions such as these: 'What are the historical roots of our understanding of the concepts and problems?' 'How are the problems addressed in different countries?' 'How are governance and its underlying conceptions connected to certain times and places?' Although these may at a first glance seem to be relativist, constructionist points of departure, they are rather the opposite: they produce concrete knowledge that contributes to answering the basic questions of what is efficient, good and right. By inquiring into the ownership of the question over time and place, the researchers have staked their own claim to ownership and the provision of answers to the most common questions in the field. As such, their work represents a reframing of addictions in Europe.

References

Beccaria, F., & Petrilli, E. (2014).The complexity of addiction: conceptions of alcohol and drug addiction among Italian scholars, 1860s–1930s. *Social History of Alcohol and Drugs*, **28**(1) 34–56.

Beccaria, F., & Rolando, S. (2013). Stakeholders' role in contemporary 'substitute drug' prescribing policies in Italy. *Substance Use & Misuse*, **48**, 943–953.

Beccaria F., & Rolando S. (2014). The Italian politics of alcohol: the creation of a public arena at the end of the 20th century. *International Journal of Drug Policies* **26**(7), 662–669

Beccaria, F., Rolando, S., Hellman, M., Bujalski, M., & Lemmens, P. (2015). From criminals to celebrities: perceptions of 'the addict' in the print press from four European countries from the nineties to today. *Substance Use & Misuse*, **50**(4), 439–453.

Berridge, V., & Mold, A. (2014). Concepts of addiction in Europe, 1860s–1930s [special issue]. *Social History of Alcohol and Drugs*, 28(1).

Berridge, V., & Mold, A. (2014). Introduction to special issue on concepts of addiction in Europe, 1860s–1930s. *Social History of Alcohol and Drugs*, 228, 4–8.

Berridge, V., Mold A., Beccaria, F., Eisenbach-Stangl, I., Herczyńska, G., Moskalewicz, J., . . . & Taylor, S. (2014). Addiction in Europe, 1860s–1960s: concepts and responses in Italy, Poland, Austria, and the United Kingdom. *Contemporary Drug Problems*, **4**(4), 551–566.

Berridge, V., Walke, J., & Mold, A. (2014). From inebriety to addiction: terminology and concepts in the UK, 1860–1930. *Social History of Alcohol and Drugs*, **28**(1) 88–106.

Blomqvist, J., & Raitasalo, K., with Melberg, H.O., Schreckenberg, D., Peschel, C., Klingemann, J., & Koski-Jännes, A. (2014). Popular images of addiction. Deliverable 3.3, Work Package 1. http://www.alicerap.eu/resources/documents.html

Bujalski, M., Moskalewicz, J., Beccaria, F., Rolando, S. Hellman, M. (2015). The depoliticization of addiction: informants in daily press reporting from three European countries in the years 1991, 1998 and 2011. Manuscript submitted for publication.

Duke, K. (forthcoming). Exchanging 'expertise' and constructing boundaries: the development of a transnational knowledge network around heroin-assisted treatment. Paper submitted to the International Journal of Drug Policy.

Duke, K., Herring, R., Thickett, A., & Thom, B. (2013). Substitution treatment in the era of 'recovery': an analysis of stakeholder roles and policy windows in Britain. *Substance Use & Misuse*, **48**, 966–976.

Duke, K., & Thom, B. (2014). The role of evidence and the expert in contemporary processes of governance: the case of opioid substitution treatment policy in England. *International Journal of Drug Policy*, **25**, 964–971.

Egerer, M. & Alanko, A. (2015). Problem gambling and the non-medical addiction model: Finnish general practitioners' and social workers' perceptions. Sosiologia. Forthcoming.

Eisenbach-Stangl, I. (2013). Deviance or innovation? Recent changes of drug substitution treatment in policy in Austria. *Substance Use & Misuse*, **48**, 1010–1021.

Eisenbach-Stangl, I. (2014). Passion and insanity: a twofold concept of addiction in Austria before World War Two. *Social History of Alcohol and Drugs*, **28**(1), 9–33

Eisenbach-Stangl, I. (2015). Toward individual responsibilities: interests at work at the major change of Austrian alcohol policy in the 1950s. Manuscript submitted for publication.

Frank, V. A., Bjerge, B., & Houborg, E. (2013). Shifts in opioid substitution treatment policy in Denmark from 2000–2011. *Substance Use & Misuse*, **48**, 997–1009.

Hellman, M. (2013). Riippuvuutta ja kompetenssia koskevat käsitykset suomalaisessa mediadiskurssissa [Perceptions of addiction and competence in Finnish media discourse]. In T. Tammi & P. Raento (Eds.), Addiktioyhteiskunta. Helsinki: Gaudeamus. 73–89.

Hellman, M. (2015, March). Addressing lifestyle-related problems: benefits from separating and joining institutional traits and adherent notions. Paper presented at the Finnish Sociology days, 15 March 2015. http://westermarck.fi/sosiologipaivat/

Hellman, M., Majamäki, M., Beccaria, F., Egerer, M., Rolando, S. Bujalski, M., & Moskalewicz, J. (2014, September). Professional images of addiction: social workers and general practitioners in three European welfare states. Deliverable 3.2 to the EU Commission, Work Package 3. ALICE RAP project. http://www.alicerap.eu/resources/documents.html

Hellman, M., Majamäki, M., Rolando, S., Bujalski, M. & Lemmens, P. (2015). What causes addiction problems? Environmental, biological and constitutional explanations in press portrayals from four European welfare societies. *Substance Use & Misuse*, **50**(4), 419–438.

Hellman, M., & Room, R. (2014). What's the story on addiction? Popular myths in the USA and Finland. *Critical Public Health*. http://www.tandfonline.com/doi/full/10.1080/09581596.2014.926308

Houborg, E., & Frank, V.A. (2014). Drug consumption rooms and the role of politics and governance in policy processes. *International Journal of Drug Policy*, **25**(5), 972–977.

Houborg, E., Frank, V.A., & Bjerge, B. (2014). From zero-tolerance to non-enforcement: creating a new space for drug policing in Copenhagen, Denmark. *Contemporary Drug Problems*, **41**(2), 261–291.

Moskalewicz, J., & Herczyńska, G. (2014). The changing meaning of addiction in Polish medical literature of the late nineteenth century and early twentieth century. *Social History of Alcohol and Drugs*, **28**(1) 57–83.

Moskalewicz, J., & Welbel, M. (2013). Walking through mud; history of the Polish methadone maintenance treatment from its stakeholders' perspective. *Substance Use & Misuse*, **48**, 977–996.

Moskalewicz, J., & Welbel, M. (2014, June). Window of opportunity open wide: changes in alcohol policy in Poland from its stakeholders' perspectives. Paper presented at 40th Annual Kettil Bruun Society Conference, Torino, 9–13 June 2014.

Sulkunen, P. (2015). The images theory of addiction. *International Journal of Alcohol and Drug Research* (early online). http://www.ijadr.org/index.php/ijadr/article/view/

Thom, B., Duke, K., Frank, V.A., & Bjerge, B. (2013). Stakeholders in opioid substitution drug user treatment policy: similarities and differences in six European countries. *Substance Use & Misuse*, **48**, 933–942.

Thom, B., Herring, R., Thickett, A., & Duke, K. (in press, 2016). The Alcohol Health Alliance: the emergence of an advocacy coalition to stimulate policy change. British Politics.

Chapter 2

Concepts of addiction in Europe in the 1970s and 1980s: what does a long view tell us about drugs, alcohol, and tobacco?

Alex Mold, Franca Beccaria, Virginia Berridge, Irmgard Eisenbach-Stangl, Grazyna Herczyńska, Jacek Moskalewicz, Enrico Petrilli, and Suzanne Taylor

2.1 Addiction concepts

Throughout history, and across Europe, an assortment of different concepts and terms were employed to describe the long-term use of illicit drugs, alcohol, and tobacco. Words such as 'inebriety', 'chronic alcohol poisoning', 'narcomania', 'dependence', and 'addiction' were used by a variety of actors in a range of contexts to describe the problems caused by psychoactive substances. In this chapter we explore some of the concepts used and the work that they did. Focusing on four European countries—Austria, Italy, Poland, and the UK—we consider the different terms applied at different times and in different places. Our key phase of analysis is the 1970s and the 1980s. These decades were important, as it was a time when illicit drug use in many countries was on the increase and new policy approaches appeared to be required to deal with an expanding population of drug users. Drawing on policy documents, including laws, regulations, decrees, government reports, and circulars, we assess the language used to describe drug, alcohol, and tobacco problems, and the nature of the policies developed to deal with them. At the same time, we endeavour to set this work in the broader context of conceptual shifts around substance use from the 1860s to the 1950s. Such a long view enables us to explore changes and continuities in the language of addiction over time as well as place.

This chapter presents findings from research conducted within Workpackage One (WP1), 'Addiction Through the Ages' of the ALICE RAP project. The aims and objectives of the ALICE RAP project, and the work of WP1, are explored in more depth in the introduction to this book. Here we detail the results of our cross-national studies, focusing on the final phase of analysis, the 1970s and 1980s. The first two stages of our work, which concentrated on the 1860s to the 1930s and the 1950s to the 1960s, are considered in greater detail in our other publications (Beccaria & Petrilli, 2014, 2015; Berridge et al., 2014; Eisenbach-Stangl, 2014a; Moskalewicz & Herczyńska, 2014), but a brief overview is provided here. Following a description of our methodology and approach, in the main body of the chapter we summarize the key developments and concepts used in alcohol, drug, and tobacco policy in Austria, Poland, Italy, and the UK during the 1970s and 1980s. From these country studies a number of key themes are extracted for further analysis, such as the differences between countries and across the substances. Finally, we conclude by reflecting on what the long history of addiction concepts in Europe tells us and what it can contribute towards current debates.

2.2 **Change over time**

Our Workpackage was tasked with assessing 'Addiction through the ages'. To explore the history of addiction concepts across Europe, we decided to focus on Austria, Italy, Poland, and the UK. This represented a good mixture of countries from different parts of Europe with varied drinking and drug-taking cultures. We wanted to gain a long view of addiction through the ages, so we decided to centre on the period from the 1860s, when alcohol and drug problems first began to attract substantial interest, up until the 1980s, when drug use expanded exponentially in many countries. We subsequently broke this period into three phases: the 1860s–1930s, the 1950s–1960s, and finally the 1970s–1980s. We agreed that as far as possible all the partners would work in the same way, to make our results more comparable.

For our first period (1860–1930), we decided that we would focus on the medical approach to substance use, and thus decided to examine one general medical journal, one specialist addiction journal, and one medical textbook for each country. We developed a list of terms used to conceptualize addiction, and then aimed to analyze the content of the medical texts and journals that we had identified over the first period. The results of this work are presented in a special issue of the journal *The Social History of Alcohol and Drugs*, and in the section of this chapter on addiction concepts in Europe, 1860s–1930s. For the second period, we decided to move away from the focus on medical texts to look at how addiction concepts were utilized within policy documents produced in the 1950s and 1960s. The rationale for this change was in part practical. The 'medical' focus of the first period had proved difficult and lengthy to operationalize for the reasons given above. Our funding and EU reporting time frames did not allow another extensive period of research. In addition, there were conceptual reasons for the change, in that our supposition was that by the 1950s, the state might be playing a greater role in the promulgation of concepts than it had done in the late nineteenth century. Privileging the medical approach might give a skewed view of the differences between countries. The results of this work are presented in more detail in an article in *Contemporary Drug Problems* and summarized in the section on addiction concepts in Europe, 1950s–1960s.

For the third phase of research, 1970s–1980s, we decided to continue with our analysis of policy documents, as this had provided a rich corpus of material. 'Policy document' proved to be an Anglocentric construct so this was broadened to encompass laws and regulations that were passed during this period. Again there were differences from one country to another with varied national traditions of policy formation and elaboration. For example, British policymaking on alcohol in this period relied on the issuing of circulars by the Ministry of Health, and we found an extensive collection of these in the National Archives (TNA), but this was not a mode used in the other countries under investigation. Nevertheless, we were able to pursue some of the same techniques. All the research partners aimed to count the number of regulations, laws, and circulars dealing with addiction, and related concepts across the substances, and also to see what language was in use. We set some broad general questions, such as:

- How do the terms used in the documents reflect or reinforce policy goals?
- Which stakeholders are behind the use of specific terms?
- What similarities and differences occur across substances and between documents?

We wanted to see if the use of terms was becoming more homogenous over time but also to identify local and national specificities. We comment on the methodological issues that arose at the end of the chapter.

2.3 Addiction concepts in Europe, 1860s–1930s

There is an extensive historiography on the development of addiction concepts, but as we point out elsewhere, the majority of this literature is confined to Britain and the United States. This has resulted in an Anglo-American interpretation of the rise of a disease-based view of drug and alcohol (and to a much lesser extent, tobacco) use since at least the late eighteenth century (Levine, 1978; Porter, 1985). Much of the literature points to a strengthening of such an approach in the nineteenth century, when medical and moral views of drug and alcohol use came together in the notion of addiction as a 'disease of the will' (Berridge, 1979; Harding, 1988; Valverde, 1997). Yet, other terms were also in circulation. In the UK and the U.S., 'inebriety' was used to describe both drink and drug problems. Continental European concepts did enter this debate through theorizing about insanity, and were applied later in the nineteenth century to alcohol and other drugs. Little attention, however, has been paid to the history of addiction concepts away from the U.S. and the UK. Our research sought to bring a European perspective to bear on the Anglo-American narrative of addiction history. Based on our analysis of addiction terms in the medical literature, a brief survey of the changing language surrounding substance use in each of the four countries points out similarities and differences with the standard view of the rise of addiction.

In Austria, two distinct sets of terminology were used to describe alcohol and drug use. The first terminology revolved around substances and their 'isms': 'alcohol' and 'alcoholism'; 'morphine' and 'morphinism'. A second set of terms concerned 'drink' and 'drunkenness'. The first terminology was rooted in the language of natural science, or *Naturwissenschaft*. This concept identified one main cause—drinking alcohol—with harmful consequences, which, after the turn of the century, increasingly included hereditary degeneration. The second terminology was a domestic language that regarded *trunksucht* (ailing because of drinking) as an incurable secondary disease of a mental disorder and at the same time as the curable consequence of passion. The two concepts coexisted, and although the first type was becoming more common within scientific work, it could neither penetrate nor replace the local concept used by German-speaking Austrians (Eisenbach-Stangl, 2014a).

A variety of terms to describe alcohol and drug use could also be found in the Italian discourse around substance use in this period. 'Alcoholic psychosis' and 'alcoholic paranoia' were in circulation, but the most commonly used concept was 'alcoholism'. Drug terms started to appear from the end of the nineteenth century, but their use was sporadic. For both drug and alcohol words, there was a divide between those concepts that emphasized the physiological, with a focus on 'poisoning', and those that centred on the pathological, such as 'morphinism', 'cocainism', and 'morphinomania'. At this time alcohol was 'owned' by positivist criminology and forensic science, and alcohol problems were often seen in eugenic terms (Beccaria & Petrilli, 2014).

During the period 1860–1930, the primary concern in Poland was with alcohol, rather than drugs or tobacco. A range of concepts was used to describe alcohol use throughout this period, such as 'alcoholism', 'drunkenness', 'poisoning' (including chronic and acute), and 'inebriety'. 'Alcoholism' gradually became the key term at the expense of others, but it meant different things at different times. 'Alcoholism' was initially conceived of as an artificially induced madness of both an acute and chronic nature. By the middle of the period, the concept of alcoholism developed to include both the medical and social consequences of drinking, and later still it was seen as a mental illness in and of itself. Another term, '*nałóg*', which linguistically could be a concept close to inebriety and/or addiction, was very rare indeed (Moskalewicz & Herczyńska, 2014). Unlike Italy, the eugenic perspective did not enter the Polish debate on alcoholism until the 1920s and 1930s.

In the UK, during the first part of the period from the 1870s to the outbreak of World War I, the term 'inebriety' appeared to dominate. Encompassing alcohol and other drugs, 'inebriety' later fell out favour, to be replaced with substance-specific terms, such as 'alcoholism'. 'Alcoholism' was present in the medical discourse since the late nineteenth century, but its use declined during the interwar years when alcohol was regarded as less of a social issue. 'Addiction', in relation to drugs but not alcohol or tobacco, was ascendant from 1918, but a range of other terms also continued to be used, especially those which were substance-specific, such as 'morphinism' (Berridge et al., 2014).

The period 1860–1930 was one of great flux across Europe with respect to the concepts used to describe drug and alcohol use. No single concept appeared to dominate; although 'alcoholism' was used in all of the countries studied, it did not necessarily mean the same thing. Local discourses, such as that around drink and the drinker in Austria, still had a role to play. After World War II, we begin to see more homogeneity around addiction terminology across Europe. For this phase of our work we analyzed the operationalization of addiction concepts in policy documents, laws, and regulations in our four countries.

2.4 **Addiction concepts in Europe, 1950s–1960s**

In Austria, the domestic terminology around drink and the drinker gave way to a more international understanding of habitual drinking. In part, this was a reflection of Austria's occupation by the Allies until 1955, meaning that the country followed America's lead, as seen in the introduction of strict laws on drugs. Addictive poisons were separated from other poisons in law, and the possession of such substances was criminalized. The actual drug problem at this time was, however, small: alcohol was a much bigger issue. This is reflected in the fact that there were more laws made at this time on alcohol (nine) than on drugs (six). Drink driving attracted legislative notice and alcohol use was established as an aggravating rather than mitigating circumstance in court cases. There was also interest in treatment, and a special system for the treatment of alcoholics was established.

In Poland, too, alcohol remained the dominant concern. Of twenty laws issued on substance use in the period, fifteen were concerned with alcohol, two dealt with illicit drugs, and three with tobacco. Early on there was some interest in drunkenness as a social problem, but when this persisted, despite the ideological presumptions of the new socialist society, the disease concept of alcoholism began to gain purchase. The notion of alcoholism reduced the problem to an individual disorder, thus shifting blame from the structural to the individual level (Moskalewicz, 1985). The first law on 'fighting alcoholism', which was passed in 1956, contained a mixture of regulatory measures, such as those relating to the availability of alcoholic beverages, alongside those aimed more at helping the user, including 'sobering up stations' and the decriminalization of public drunkenness. Alcohol at this time was regarded as both a medical and a social problem; the approaches were combined in the introduction of compulsory treatment. Little attention was paid to drugs apart from restrictions on access to certain substances and the registration of drug 'abusers'. Interest in tobacco was confined to the prohibition of smoking in some public places such as buses and sporting events.

In contrast, in Italy during the 1950s and 1960s, there was much more emphasis on drugs rather than alcohol. Although Italy also established specialized treatment centres for 'social diseases', of which 'toxicosis' from narcotics was one, Italian substance use policy at this time concentrated on drugs and associated crime. This is reflected in the laws that were passed: nine laws on drugs, eight on alcohol, and three on tobacco. The laws on alcohol and tobacco were concerned predominantly with production, taxation, and trade—there were no references to abuse or addiction. In terms of problems relating to substance use, the focus was very much on drugs. In the first part of the period, the primary concern was the new synthetic analgesics such as Dolantin. Later in the 1950s, there was more interest in Italy's role in the international drug trade, especially in relation to corruption and the country's apparent slowness to deal with traffickers.

Policy in the UK was also especially concerned with drugs, although there was emphasis on drug treatment as well as drug-related crime. In the period studied, the majority of laws passed were on drugs (39), compared to tobacco (8) and alcohol (6). Other kinds of policy documents, such as Ministry of Health circulars, also tended to centre on drugs, with thirty-eight being issued on drugs, compared to twenty-six on tobacco and five on alcohol. Not all of these related to 'addiction', though, and some laws, such as the Dangerous Drugs Act of 1951, were framed by international commitments. An attempt to define 'addiction' was made by the Interdepartmental Committee on Heroin Addiction in 1961, a definition that was subsequently used in legislation. Other measures included the establishment of treatment centres for heroin addicts. A treatment system also developed for alcoholics. Tobacco was not seen in terms of addiction at this time, with policy instead emphasizing public education about the health dangers of smoking rather than the disease of addiction.

Looking across the different countries, we can see a coming-together of concepts around 'alcoholism' and 'addiction', although other terms were still in circulation. International influences were also becoming more apparent, but at the same time national differences remained. There was, for instance, a differing emphasis on drugs and alcohol between countries. Moreover, not all of the laws and policy documents produced in this period focused on the 'addictive' nature of substances. In relation to other health risks tobacco was of relatively little interest, except in terms of trade, and in the UK. To what extent did such patterns continue into the 1970s and 1980s?

2.5 **Addiction concepts in Austria, 1970s–1980s**

In Austria, alcohol was a minor policy issue during the 1970s and 1980s. There were no laws made specifically on alcohol at this time, although alcohol did appear in other pieces of legislation. There were, for instance, regulations issued on the use of alcohol in the workplace in 1972, but this was part of a broader law concerned with health and safety (*Arbeitnehmerschutzgesetz* [Law on the Protection of Life, Health and Morals of Employees], 1972). There was also interest in the wine trade, especially following an adulteration scandal in 1985 when antifreeze was found in Austrian wine (Eisenbach-Stangl, 1992). The only piece of legislation that concerned alcohol directly was a ban on advertising for spirits and tobacco on public broadcasting services, introduced in 1974 (*Bundesgesetz Über Die Errichtung Und Die Aufgaben Des Österreichischen Rundfunk* [Law on Public Serving Broadcasting], 1974). The addictive properties of alcohol did not appear to attract legislative interest at this time, and as a result, the terminology used in the laws tended to emphasize the short-term effects of alcohol, such as 'drunkenness' and 'intoxication', rather than 'alcoholism'.

Conversely, the law around drugs was much more focused on addiction and its effects. In the period 1970–1980, seven laws were passed that concerned '*Suchgift*' or 'addictive poisons'. Legislation dealt with both drug treatment and drug control. A law passed in 1980, for instance, established drug treatment facilities providing 'therapy instead of punishment' as well as treatment obligations for drug users, instigated reporting obligations for health facilities and other organizations, and formulated a health education programme (*Suchtgiftgesetznovelle* [Amendment of Penal Side Law/Drug Law], 1980). Such developments in drug policy at this time reflected an increase in drug consumption in the 1970s, but also changing patterns of drug use. Iatrogenic drugs began to be replaced with heroin, and by the 1980s the user population became increasingly socially marginalized (Eisenbach-Stangl, 2000; Pilgram, 1980). More widely, broader political changes in Austria resulted in a less paternalistic approach to government and these were reflected in a drug policy that decriminalized possession for personal use and emphasized treatment rather than prosecution. In the 1970s, drug treatment was mostly abstinence-oriented, but by the 1980s more emphasis was placed on harm reduction, especially after the appearance of AIDS (Eisenbach-Stangl, 2014b). On the other hand, police powers increased, and convicted drug dealers met with long sentences. Such a dichotomy in policy was not only about domestic politics—it also had an international dimension. The location of the UN Office on Drugs and Crime in Vienna from 1980, and the city's hosting of the meetings of the International Narcotics Board, made legislators keen to ensure that Austria abided by all international treaties on drugs.

If drugs were a major policy issue in Austria during the 1970s and 1980s, the same cannot be said of tobacco. There was, of course, the ban on tobacco advertising on public broadcasting as there was for spirits, and in 1983 employees also got the right to work in a smoke-free environment (*Allgemeine Arbeitnehmerschutzverordnung* [Decree on the Protection of Life, Health and Morals of Employees, Replacing Previous Regulations], 1983). Outpatient treatment for those wishing to stop smoking was introduced in 1980, but the laws on tobacco did not refer to this in terms of 'addiction'. So, by the end of the 1980s, the picture across the substances was diverse: alcohol legislation tended to focus on the effects of drinking rather than alcoholism, drug policy was divided between treatment and control approaches, and tobacco smoking was not seen as an addiction.

2.6 Addiction concepts in Italy, 1970s–1980s

Italian alcohol policy in this period, like that of Austria, was primarily concerned with the regulation of production and trade rather than the effects of alcohol consumption. Laws on alcohol passed between 1970 and the end of the 1980s dealt with the taxation of alcoholic beverages and the wine market; the Parliament was critical of European policies that would have had a negative impact on the Italian wine trade (Law No. 408, 1984; Motion 3, 1968; Motion 4, 1969; Motion 93, 1971). Alcohol treatment was mentioned in a law introduced in 1975, but the primary focus of this piece of legislation was illegal drugs (Law No. 685, 1975).

Indeed, as had been the case in the 1950s and 1960s, illicit drugs generated by far the most legislative interest in Italy. Drug policy in the 1970s and 1980s was characterized by heterogeneous discourses: prevention, care, public order, social concern, and international relationships all played a part. Like many other European countries, Italy experienced a boom in cannabis use from the mid-1960s and an increase in opiate use from the early 1970s. In response, a law was introduced in 1975 that made a distinction between drug dealers and users, and also encouraged treatment for 'addicts', who were defined as sick people in need of help (Law No. 685, 1975). In 1979, a motion was introduced which called upon the government to take action to combat the problem of 'tossicomania' (addiction) among prison inmates (Motion 16, 1979). Towards the end of the 1980s, legislation on drug taking and driving came into force, and there was a decree that made provisions aimed at reducing the risk of HIV infection (Law No. 111, 1988; Decree-Law No. 14, 1988). But, as in the earlier period, more attention was devoted to control of the drug trade than the consequences of drug use. The role of the Mafia in national and international drug trafficking was of particular concern, generating laws, reports, and motions in Parliament (Commission of Inquiry's Report, 1976; Law No. 743, 1981; Motion 172, 1986).

Once more, tobacco seemed to cause less anxiety amongst Italian lawmakers than other substances. A law was passed in 1975 that prohibited smoking in certain places such as on public transport, but, as with alcohol, most legislation focused on production and trade (Law No. 584, 1975). This raises an interesting contrast between alcohol and tobacco policy on the one hand and drug policy on the other, something that was further underscored by Italy's relationship with international regulations in this area. The Italian legislature was content to follow all international requirements with respect to illicit drugs, but not on alcohol or tobacco, which were important to the Italian economy.

2.7 Addiction concepts in Poland, 1970s–1980s

A different approach to addiction can be found in Poland during the 1970s and 1980s. Here, the focus was very much on alcohol, which generated by far the most legislation in this period, with forty-five regulations as opposed to nine on drugs and just two on tobacco. Alcohol regulation spanned a variety of topics, including treatment, drink driving, and drinking in the workplace. A major piece of legislation was the Law on Upbringing in Sobriety and Counteracting Alcoholism, passed in 1982. The text of the law used a variety of terms to describe alcohol problems, including 'alcoholism', 'alcohol abuse', and 'alcohol dependence'. The law stated that a 'citizens' life in sobriety is a necessary condition of the moral and material well-being of the Nation'; its purpose was to establish a comprehensive system of alcohol prevention, control, and treatment

(Law on Upbringing in Sobriety and Counteracting Alcoholism, 1982). This system was to involve public bodies and the voluntary sector as well as the Catholic church and other religious denominations. The law also introduced strict control measures, most notably, a state monopoly on the distribution of alcoholic drinks for off-premise sales, an approach based on the Nordic model. This system was later dismantled in the transition to a market economy.

Beneath the legislative changes, important conceptual shifts were also taking place. These can be detected in the language used in the laws to describe alcohol problems. A militaristic rhetoric of 'fighting alcoholism' was gradually replaced with more moderate terms such as 'counteracting' alcoholism. Greater precision was also introduced to the legislation, with the vague term 'insobriety' being replaced with a more exact definition based on blood-alcohol content levels. The terms used to describe individuals with alcohol problems also changed, as 'alcoholics' became 'alcohol dependents'—a development that underscored the supposed medical sources of the problem. A concept of 'compulsory treatment' adopted twenty-five years earlier was replaced by a so-called 'obligation to undertake treatment' which could be imposed by a court. 'Obliged' persons had to admit themselves to treatment or otherwise be brought by the police to a treatment centre, although they were free to leave treatment at any time. In this way medical services offering alcohol treatment were liberated from providing involuntary treatment (Moskalewicz & Wald, 1987). The term 'alcoholism' was still in use, but it referred to the social phenomenon of excessive drinking or the social problems connected with alcohol use, rather than those of the individual drinker.

A similar approach can be found in Polish drug policy in this period. The language used in the legislation appeared to reflect a nonpunitive approach to drug-using individuals, who were referred to as 'drug-dependent persons'. But 'drug abuse' or 'narcomania' was used to describe the social phenomenon of drug taking. The Law on Preventing Drug Addiction, passed in 1985, set out measures to reduce drug supplies, prevent the spread of drug use, and treat addicts. The law decriminalized drug possession for individual users, but at the same time introduced compulsory drug treatment for underaged drug-dependent persons. Control of young drug users was thus to be achieved through treatment rather than prosecution.

Treatment, however, was not an issue referred to in relation to tobacco. Indeed, smoking appeared to be of little concern to Polish legislators. The 1970s witnessed only one piece of legislation on tobacco; namely, the Ordinance of the Minister of Health and Social Welfare of 1974 on Limiting Smoking in Regard to Health, which banned smoking in a few public places and introduced smoke-free areas in others, such as designated train compartments and non-smoking rooms in restaurants. Fifteen years later, on the eve of wider political and economic transformations, the Law on Economic Activity of 1988 removed the state monopoly on tobacco and opened up the market to the private sector. Once again, tobacco seemed to encounter a different response than either alcohol or drugs in this period.

2.8 Addiction concepts in the UK, 1970s–1980s

The relative neglect of tobacco in Poland, Italy, and Austria during the 1970s and 1980s was not a pattern replicated in the UK. Of the thirty-four major policy documents (including government reports and circulars, as well as laws), fourteen were concerned with tobacco, nine with alcohol, and eleven with drugs. Legislation on tobacco dealt with tax and duty as it had done in the past, but in this period taxation was also being used in an attempt to curb tobacco consumption. Such a move was rooted in a policy context that not only emphasized the harm smoking posed to health, but was also concerned with the properties of tobacco itself. In 1971, the Royal College of Physicians (RCP) report, 'Smoking and Health', referred to 'dependence' on tobacco (Royal College of Physicians, 1971). 'Dependence' was, of course, a concept that had already been used in British drug and alcohol policy, but its use in relation to tobacco was a new development.

'Dependence' was a term still seen occasionally in alcohol policy documents in the 1970s and 1980s, but a variety of other concepts were also in play. Alcohol 'misuse', 'abuse', 'alcoholism', and 'alcohol-related harm' were all present, and a new term, 'problem drinker', came on the scene. 'Problem drinking' was seen as being both a disease and a social problem (Department of Health, 1973). 'Excessive drinking' was a term sometimes used interchangeably with 'problem drinking' (Department of Health and Social Security, 1977; Department of Health, 1981). Although some laws concerning alcohol were introduced during this period—such as the *Road Traffic Act, 1972*, which made it an offence to drive under the influence of alcohol, as well as laws which banned drinking at, and when travelling to, certain sports events—alcohol policy tended to be made through reports and departmental circulars (Road Traffic Act, 1972). Government reports and those by professional bodies, like the Royal College of Physicians, encouraged the development of treatment services for individuals with alcohol problems, but also began to emphasize the wider dangers that alcohol could pose to the health of the population. By the mid-1980s, there was interest in encouraging 'sensible drinking' based on the quantification of alcoholic drink consumption in 'units' (Department of Health, 1981; Royal College of Physicians, 1987).

Some of the same concepts used in alcohol policy in this period also appeared in drug policy in the UK. Drug 'dependence' was a term still in operation, and a key piece of legislation, which brought in the contemporary classification of illegal drugs into three categories, Class A, B, and C, with differing legal penalties attached, was concerned with drug 'misuse'. In 1982, the government's Advisory Committee on Drug Misuse published a report, *Treatment and Prevention*, which referred to the 'problem drug taker'. Like the 'problem drinker', the 'problem drug taker' was not only an individual with a disease, but someone 'who experiences social, psychological, physical or legal problems related to intoxication and/or regular excessive consumption and/or dependence as a consequence of his own use of drugs' (Advisory Council on the Misuse of Drugs, 1982, p. 34). Unlike alcohol, however, there was no concept of 'sensible' drug taking, although there were efforts to attempt to reduce the harm that drug users could cause both to themselves and to society, an approach that strengthened in the wake of HIV/AIDS. This did not necessarily result in a more liberal drug policy; although drug treatment became somewhat more flexible, from 1985 onwards, government strategy documents tended to emphasize control of the drug trade rather than the regulation of drug treatment (Mold, 2008).

2.9 **Key themes**

What do these country case studies tell us when viewed collectively? It is clear that there was some fluctuation around the various terms used to describe drug, alcohol, and tobacco use both within the different countries and over time. We can observe the introduction of new terminologies, such as 'problem drinker/drug taker' in the UK and 'drug dependence' in Poland. At the same time, older concepts, such as 'alcoholism', persisted. The meaning behind the terms used to describe substance use also varied. Some of this language suggested a disease-based approach, such as 'dependence', whereas others hinted more at the social consequences of substance use, like 'alcohol abuse' and 'drug misuse'. Even supposedly medicalized terms, like 'alcoholism', could, as in the case of Poland, continue to encompass both the medical and the social consequences of drinking. It is also interesting to observe where the language of addiction was not used. 'Dependence' was a term beginning to be applied to tobacco in the UK, but it did not appear in any of the other countries studied. Despite such variations, there did appear to be greater stability around the use of key terms such as 'dependence' across the different countries than there had been in the first phase (1860–1930). As in the second period (1950s–1960s), there seemed to be some degree of coherence around the language of addiction even if variations and modifications continued to appear.

Such an increase in homogeneity could be related to international influences. The roles played by the World Health Organization (WHO) expert committees on drugs, alcohol, and tobacco are discussed in more detail elsewhere in this volume (Chapter 4); there are signs that the work of such bodies influenced the domestic framing of substance use. In the UK, for instance, the definition of alcoholism used in a Department of Health circular on the provision of services for alcoholics in 1973 drew explicitly on that provided by the WHO (Department of Health, 1973). The global framework designed to regulate illegal drugs, alcohol, and tobacco had other effects, too. In Austria, the location of the UN Office on Drugs and Crime in Vienna not only ensured that the country abided by all the international regulations on narcotics control, but also added impetus to the efforts of those who wanted to introduce stricter measures to domestic policy. Elsewhere, however, international pressures could be resisted. Italy, for instance, was reluctant to accept global regulation of alcohol and tobacco, as both substances were important to the national economy. Yet, at the same time, international concerns were at the heart of Italy's drug policy. Not only did Italy sign up (as did all of the countries under investigation) to the United Nations' Single Convention on Narcotic Drugs in 1961, but the country's role in the transnational illegal drug trade was also a major political and policy issue.

Indeed, despite the homogenizing effect of international governance in some areas, considerable national variation in drug, alcohol, and tobacco policies remained. This can be seen in the balance of policy documents produced by the various nations across the substances. In the UK, Italy, and Austria, there was more legislative emphasis on drugs, whereas in Poland there was greater stress placed on alcohol. Such discrepancies could be the result of the differing scale and nature of the drug use and trade in the respective countries at this time, with the UK, Italy, and Austria experiencing more drug-related problems than Poland. Contrasting policy emphasis also translated into some differences in policy. Poland and Austria decriminalized personal drug possession, whereas Italy and the UK did not, although both countries did distinguish in law between drug dealing and drug possession.

The case study nations also responded to alcohol differently. Italy wanted to avoid restriction of the wine trade, whereas Poland introduced a state monopoly on the sale of alcohol. Austrian legislation at this time was only tangentially concerned with alcohol, and although on the surface the same appeared to be true of the UK, alcohol policy there was made more through reports produced by expert committees and government departments than by acts of parliament.

Tobacco smoking seemed to be an issue of little concern in all of the countries except the UK. Indeed, Britain was the only country to view tobacco as potentially dependence-producing in this period. The UK was also the first of our case study nations to start to take significant action against smoking, perhaps because some key research on tobacco harm had been conducted there (Berridge, 2007).

The differences between countries and their substance use policies were a reflection of the different problems that they faced, but such contrasts also pointed to specificities in national politics and the policymaking process. Polish alcohol policy was a reflection not only of the need to deal with alcohol, but was also rooted in conflict between the state and the unions. The alcohol debate initiated in the 1970s was reinvigorated at the beginning of the 1980s in a hectic conflict between the authorities and independent trade union movements, which under the banner of Solidarity exploited the alcohol question as a political weapon in their fight for moral supremacy. Blaming the political authorities for pushing alcohol in order to increase budget revenues and to more easily manipulate the drunken society represented in fact an attempt to discredit the ruling party and deprive it of the moral credentials to remain in power (Moskalewicz, 1981; Bielewicz & Moskalewicz, 1982). Eventual consensus on restrictive alcohol legislation indicated shaky prospects for turning down political conflict. In contrast, the drug debate avoided open antagonization of both sides of the political conflict. Drug abuse was defined as an expression of intergenerational conflict, and therefore a therapeutic community approach seemed to be a more appropriate solution than any revolutionary changes in power distribution (Świątkiewicz et al., 1998). Liberal drug legislation adopted in the mid-1980s was to herald the withdrawal of military rule and was a step towards a more democratic civic order.

In Austria, broader changes in the nature of politics during this period also influenced the direction of drug policy. A move away from a strict, hierarchical, patriarchal structure towards a more egalitarian mode with greater rights for women and children resulted in more tolerance of the 'socially deviant'. As a result, drug laws became more liberal, with greater emphasis on treatment rather than punishment. In Italy, concern about corruption, the Mafia, and the international drug trade meant that policy was outward- as well as inward-facing. British substance use policy was a reflection of the country's pragmatic system of government, where policy tended to be made less through laws and more through expert reports and government departmental circulars. National differences in policy were thus the result of national circumstances as well as other influences.

2.10 The long view

Taking the long view, we can observe the rise of a plethora of terms to describe alcohol and drug problems in the nineteenth and early twentieth century. Many of these fell away by the second half of the twentieth century, with some coherence forming around key terms such as 'dependence' and 'addiction'. Yet other terms continued to exist, and some new concepts also came on the scene. To some extent these were country- and time-specific, as with the brief career of 'problem drinker/drug taker' in the UK. Whatever the word used, however, there seemed to be a dual dimension to substance use terminology. On the one hand, there was a concept that emphasized the disease-based nature of substance use, whereas on the other hand, there were terms that stressed the social effects of drinking or drug taking. Sometimes these elements were encapsulated in separate words like 'drug misuse' versus 'drug addiction', but sometimes the term meant both a disease that needed to be treated and a social problem that required control. Such a dichotomy is also reflected in substance use policies which have tended to have the twin aims of helping those with drug and alcohol problems and mitigating the effect that these have on wider society. Once more, the emphasis between these different elements changes over time and place, but both can usually be found.

The long view of addiction concepts in Austria, Italy, Poland, and the UK therefore has much to add to current debates. By pointing out the continuities and changes between countries and at different times, we can tease out more general trends. Although a degree of stability has been achieved around addiction concepts, these still encapsulate a variety of meanings that translate into different treatment and policy approaches. By understanding the history of such concepts, and how and why they came into and out of use, we can better understand addiction terminology and substance use policy today.

References

Advisory Council on the Misuse of Drugs. (1982).Treatment and rehabilitation. London: HMSO.

Allgemeine Arbeitnehmerschutzverordnung [Decree on the Protection of Life, Health and Morals of Employees, Replacing Previous Regulations]. (1983).

Arbeitnehmerschutzgesetz [Law on the Protection of Life, Health and Morals of Employees]. (1972).

Beccaria, F., & Petrilli, E. (2014). The complexity of addiction: different conceptualizations of alcohol and drug addiction(s) among Italian scholars in the late 19th and early 20th century. *Social History of Alcohol and Drugs*, **28**(1), 34–56.

Beccaria, F., & Petrilli, E. (2015). The Italian 'alcohol question' from 1860 to 1930: two opposing scientific interpretations. *International Journal of Alcohol and Drug Research* **4**(1), 37–43.

Berridge, V. (1979). Morality and medical science: concepts of narcotic addiction in Britain, 1820–1926. *Annals of Science*, **36**, 67–85.

Berridge, V. (2007). Marketing health: smoking and the discourse of public health in Britain, 1945–2000. Oxford: Oxford University Press.

Berridge, V., Mold, A., Beccaria, F., Herczyńska, G., Moskalewicz, J., Petrilli, E., & Taylor, S. (2014). Addiction in Europe, 1860s–1960s: concepts and responses in Italy, Poland, Austria and the United Kingdom. *Contemporary Drug Problems* **41**(4) 551–566.

Berridge, V., Mold, A., & Walke, J. (2014). From inebriety to addiction: terminology and concepts in the UK, 1860–1930. *Social History of Alcohol and Drugs*, 28(1), 88–106.

Bielewicz, A., & Moskalewicz, J. (1982). Temporary prohibition: the Gdańsk experience, August 1980. *Contemporary Drug Problems*, **11**, 367–381.

Bundesgesetz Über Die Errichtung Und Die Aufgaben Des Österreichischen Rundfunk [Law on Public Serving Broadcasting]. (1974).

Commission of Inquiry's Report. (1976).

Decree-Law No. 14. (1988).

Department of Health. (1973). Community services for alcoholics. London. HMSO.

Department of Health. (1981). Prevention and health: drinking sensibly. London: HMSO.

Department of Health and Social Security. (1977). Advisory Committee on Alcoholism. Report on prevention. London: HMSO.

Eisenbach-Stangl, I. (1992). Der Österreichische Weinskandal von 1985 Und Seine Folgen. *Wiener Zeitschrift Für Suchtforschung*, **4**, 3–10.

Eisenbach-Stangl, I. (2000). Silly junkies: Aussteiger, Kriminelle, Kranke? Zuschreibungen Und Lebensrealitäten. In G. Schinnerl & P. Neubauer (Eds.), Perspektiven Der Drogenarbeit Und Drogenpolitik. Wien: Ein Lesebuch, Verein der Wiener Sozialprojekte. 22–27.

Eisenbach-Stangl, I. (2014a). Passion and insanity: a twofold concept of addiction in Austria before World War Two. *Social History of Alcohol and Drugs*, **28**(1), 9–33.

Eisenbach-Stangl, I. (2014b). Deviance or innovation? Recent changes of drug substitution treatment policy in Austria. *Substance Use & Misuse*, **48**, 1010–1021.

Harding, G. (1988). Opiate addiction morality and medicine: from moral illness to pathological disease. Basingstoke: Macmillan.

Levine, H.G. (1978). The discovery of addiction: changing conceptions of habitual drunkenness in America. *Journal of Studies on Alcohol*, **39**, 143–174.

Mold, A. (2008). Heroin: the treatment of addiction in twentieth-century Britain. De Kalb: Northern Illinois University Press.

Moskalewicz, J. (1981). Alcohol as a public issue: recent developments in alcohol control in Poland. *Contemporary Drug Problems*, **10**, 11–21.

Moskalewicz, J. (1985). The monopolization of the alcohol arena by the state. *Contemporary Drug Problems*, **12**, 117–128.

Moskalewicz, J., & Herczyńska, G. (2014). The changing meaning of addiction in Polish medical literature of the late nineteenth century and early twentieth century. *Social History of Alcohol and Drugs*, **28**(1), 57–87.

Moskalewicz, J., & Wald, I. (1987). From compulsory treatment to the obligation to undertake treatment: conceptual evolution in Poland. *Contemporary Drug Problems*, **14**, 39–51.

Ordinance of the Minister of Health and Social Welfare on Limiting Smoking in Regard to Health. (1974).

Pilgram, A. (1980). Suchtgiftkriminalität in Österreich—Anleitung Zur Unvoreingenommenen Lektüre Amtlicher Statisken. In R. Mader & H. Strozka (Eds.), Drogenpolitik Zwischen Therapie Und Strafe, Jugend Und Volk. Wien. 203–233.

Porter, R. (1985). The drinking man's disease: the 'pre-history' of alcoholism in Georgian Britain. *British Journal of Addiction*, **80**, 385–396.

Road Traffic Act. (1972).

Royal College of Physicians. (1971). Smoking and health now: a new report and summary on smoking and its effects on health. London: Pitman.

Royal College of Physicians. (1987). A great and growing evil: the medical consequences of alcohol abuse. London: Tavistock.

Suchtgiftgesetznovelle [Amendment of Penal Side Law/drug Law]. (1980).

Świątkiewicz, G., Moskalewicz, J., & Sierosławski, J. (1998). Therapeutic communities as a major response to drug abuse in Poland. In G. Hunt (Ed.), Drug treatment systems in an international perspective: drugs, demons and delinquents. London: Sage. 124–132.

Valverde, M. (1997). 'Slavery from within': the invention of alcoholism and the question of free will. *Social History*, **22**(3), 251–268.

Chapter 3

Concepts and policies directed at drug use in Denmark, Finland, and Sweden

Bagga Bjerge, Esben Houborg, Johan Edman, and Riikka Perälä

3.1 Conceptualization and management of drug-related concerns

This chapter undertakes a comparative analysis of how drug users and drug use are conceptualized and managed in Denmark, Finland, and Sweden. Although the Nordic countries are often described as quite similar welfare states (Baldwin, 1990; Esping-Andersen, 1990 Lehto, 1994), this chapter demonstrates that similar political systems can adopt different policies directed at similar conditions. More specifically, the chapter explores the following questions:

- How do welfare states that are normally perceived as similar sometimes adopt highly divergent policies towards similar conditions?
- How can we analytically and empirically understand differences in conceptualizing and managing drug use and drug users in Denmark, Finland, and Sweden?

Inspired by welfare regime research (e.g. Baldwin, 1990; Esping-Andersen, 1990), we employ the concept of *policy space*. This approach is based on work by Benoit (2003) and Dorn (1995), who view drug policy as part of societal management of risks along with other policy areas (cf. Houborg & Bjerge, 2011). The management of risk may be influenced by various ideologies. Benoit (2003) emphasizes political and institutional history as an important factor in the development of drug policies: a history of either socializing or individualizing risks as collective or individual responsibilities, respectively, influences the extent to which drug policy emphasizes control and welfare strategies. Dorn (1995) distinguishes between different governmental discourses that may affect drug policies. Following Rose (1999), the idea of *political rationalities* is included in our understanding of policy spaces. Political rationalities are ways of constructing reality as amenable to intervention and ways of thinking about how government should be exercised (Rose, 1999, p. 42). Studying policy from the perspective of political rationalities implies focusing on (1) where, how, and by whom particular phenomena are constructed as requiring management; (2) the kinds of concepts used to explain these phenomena, and who acquires the authority to speak the truth about them; (3) the methods, measures, and technologies that are deployed to handle the phenomena; and (4) the kinds of truths and authorities to which individuals and groups must be subjected in order to be accepted as particular kinds of subjects.

In order to explore similarities and differences between Danish, Finnish, and Swedish drug policy, we present an overview of each country's drug policy history and analyze how different concepts and policies have evolved. We subsequently examine three topics that have given rise to debate in all three countries; these topics are thus well suited for an investigation into how particular political rationalities have come to dominate drug policies: sanctions against drug users, coercive treatment, and medical substitution treatment.

3.2 **Overview of drug policy history and concepts in Denmark, Finland, and Sweden**

3.2.1 **Denmark**

In Denmark, the term *misbrug* has been used since the 1870s, when non-medical use of drugs first became an object of intervention. *Misbrug* can mean both 'misuse' and 'abuse'. The word has taken on various nuances over time. The term was initially mainly used with respect to non-medical use of drugs and was thus not necessarily associated with behavioural problems, although it was sometimes also used to mean 'abuse', indicating such problems. Closely related to the meaning of 'non-medical use' is the legal meaning of *misbrug* as 'illegal use', particularly after Denmark criminalized unauthorized possession of controlled drugs in 1955. Since the late 1960s, *misbrug* has mainly been used to mean 'abuse', and it has been the most common term in political, professional, and popular discourse concerning behavioural problems in relation to drugs. The term *afhængighed*, which can mean both 'addiction' and 'dependency', has also been widely used since the 1870s, though less so than *misbrug*. In certain contexts, distinctions have been made between *misbrug* and *afhængighed*, especially in professional and scientific discourse. Since the 1870s, other concepts have been used, but much less frequently than *misbrug* and *afhængighed*. One term is *tilvænning*, which can be translated as 'learning a habit' or 'getting used to' but can also imply physical addiction. Another term is *forfaldenhed*, which means something like a 'bad habit'. *Narkomani* ('narcomania') is also a term that has been used from the 1930s. The term was originally used within the scientific community to designate dependence on opiates but was later—particularly since the 1970s—popularized as almost interchangeable with *misbrug*. It is thus still common to call a person with drug problems a *narkoman* (narcomaniac) in popular discourse.

In Denmark, non-medical use of drugs emerged as an object of intervention by the medical community in the 1870s and 1880s, with inspiration drawn from other countries and particularly the work of Levinstein in Germany. The issue was closely related to misuse (non-medical use) of morphine; problems that could develop in association with this were labelled 'morphinism' (Houborg, 2014). In 1883, the Danish doctor Knud Pontoppidan published his treatise on *The Chronic Morphinism*, which became the central reference for discussions about drugs well into the 1940s. Pontoppidan concluded that morphinism was developed by predisposed individuals primarily due to psychopathology. In his view, the most important measures to apply were a vigilant medical practice and strict rules to prevent such people from developing a pathological 'hunger' for the drug.

During the 1880s, the Royal College of Medicine issued more restrictive prescription rules. 'Chronic morphinism' was thus seen and regulated as a medical issue and an individual problem. The introduction of new drugs, particularly amphetamine in the 1930s, led to the introduction of the general term 'euphomania' to designate the development of a pathological craving for and dependence on drugs. This concept was developed at the Institute for Pharmacology, University of Copenhagen, to designate a pathological craving for the euphoric rather than the narcotic effect of the drugs (Møller, 1945). The term 'euphomania' became the key term in the 1950s and 1960s. In the late 1940s, the first drug scene developed in Denmark, in which groups of people would interact around acquiring, exchanging, and using drugs (Houborg, 2010; Nimb, 1972). The drug scene came to the attention of the police, and the drug problem transcended the medical institution as a matter of regulation: it became a social as well as an individual problem. It was to a great degree the desire on the part of the police to control the new drug scene that led to the introduction of legislation in 1955 criminalizing possession of illicit drugs for personal use (Jepsen, 2008; Storgaard, 2000).

During the 1960s, a new drug scene emerged, associated with the new youth culture. A rapid development of drug experimentation among young Danes made drug use an important policy issue in the 1960s and early 1970s (Houborg, 2008; Houborg & Vammen, 2012; Storgaard, 2000). The new phenomenon was initially called *ungdomsnarkomanien* (the youth narcomania), but in the 1960s *narkomani* was gradually displaced by the term *misbrug*, here meaning 'abuse'.

An important reason for this was that sociological conceptions of drug problems came to dominate discussions (Houborg, 2008). Closely related to the conceptualization of 'drug abuse' as socially learned, 'drug abuse' also came to be seen as a 'social problem' rather than an individual moral and/or mental problem. This was because young people who developed problems with drugs often came from a background of social deprivation and/or other social problems. 'Drug abuse' came to be seen as a symptom of more structural problems in Danish society (Houborg, 2008). To control the supply of drugs, harsher sanctions were introduced for violations of the drug laws prohibiting drug trafficking and drug distribution. However, parliament made the passing of the legislation conditional upon drug users not being exposed to harsher punishment. Possession of illicit drugs for personal use was thus decriminalized through a circular put out by the attorney general ordering police and prosecutors not to press charges for possession in most cases.

The medical system found it difficult to handle young drug users. A new drug treatment system was developed based on a conception of 'drug use' as meaningful, socially learned behaviour—mainly among socially deprived young people. This social conception of drug use meant that methadone maintenance treatment (MMT) was rejected as medicalization of a social problem (Houborg, 2013). Because many people with drug problems were not in drug treatment in the 1980s, there was a partial reconceptualization of the drug problem so that it became a matter of social exclusion. To assist this group, the conception of harm reduction was introduced into Danish drug policy, thereby opening up MMT (Frank et al., 2013). In 2004, the Danish parliament repealed the decriminalization of possession of illicit drugs for personal use that had existed since 1969. From 2004, Denmark has therefore had a zero-tolerance policy on possession of illicit drugs, and only dependent drug users with very few economic resources are exempt from punishment. In 2007, heroin maintenance treatment was introduced, followed by drug consumption facilities in 2012. This means that today Denmark on the one hand has a drug policy that places more emphasis on control and sanctions of drug users than before, but on the other hand has a rather elaborate harm reduction and welfare-oriented policy.

3.2.2 Finland

In Finland, drug use and drug users have been defined and conceptualized primarily within two frameworks: the medical and the criminal. The medical framework dominated from the 1930s until the end of World War II. From the 1950s until the turn of the millennium, the criminal framework was central, with the police being the key experts. In the 1990s, the role of medicine and doctors once again gained prominence, leading to new 'brain-based' interpretations of drug problems and discussions about the 'medicalization' of the Finnish drug question. This was accompanied by the appearance of novel problematizations, including harm reduction, leading to new ways of thinking and talking about drug problems.

Pekka Hakkarainen (1992) has compressed the formulation of drug problems in Finland into a narrative. The story starts in the 1930s, with descriptions of a small number of opioid misusers in Helsinki. This use, referred to as 'upper class morphinism' in the subsequent research (e.g. Jaakkola 1969) took place in small circles, and the substances used (typically morphine) were obtained from pharmacies. No criminal activities were involved, and no burden was placed on social and health services. Many users had a wealthy and educated background. The largest user groups were doctors and other healthcare professionals, followed by artists engaging in a 'bohemian' lifestyle. The police had no specific interest in controlling drug use, and apart from a few speculative articles in the press about the spread of cocaine, drug use was of little interest to the media. The main frameworks for dealing with drug use were medical and individual, and doctors were regarded as the main experts if problems occurred (Partanen, 2002).

During and after World War II, the number of drug users began increasing, coupled with changes in users' social backgrounds as well as in the substances used. Morphine was replaced by heroin, which had become a widely used painkiller and cough medicine during the war; for instance, among soldiers. Drug problems started to be seen, in fact, as synonymous with heroin use, so that, for example, it was typical to refer to a drug user as a 'heroinist' or 'heroin user' (Hakkarainen, 1992, p. 55). Other commonly used terms were 'narcomaniac' and 'euphomaniac' (ibid.). The use of terminology was not, however, particularly coherent or accurate. No differentiation was made between experimentation, use, and addiction, and one could speak of 'narcomania' already after a single instance of use.

The main difference with the situation before the war was that the new users came from the working class and had a background in criminal subcultures. The drug use also became more visible in a societal sense: it took place outdoors and in large groups more and more often and caused public commotion. Police became the most prominent experts. The press started calling for more active police surveillance and improvements in drug legislation, and the police used the press to advance its own agenda; for instance, by taking journalists along on drug raids (Hakkarainen, 1992, p. 104). Eventually, prescription policies were tightened, and heroin was removed from the pharmacopoeia (Oksanen, 2008). By the 1950s, heroin use had subsided, and the prevalence of drug use dropped to the same level as before the war. By the beginning of the 1960s, heroin had been replaced by methadone, and a new criminal subculture was formed around its use. The problem was, however, considered quite marginal.

With the 1960s came cannabis use. This period has been regarded as the 'first drug wave', resulting in a heated and morally loaded public discussion in the media about the risks of drug use as well the adoption of various preventive measures (Hakkarainen, 1992; Partanen, 2002; Salasuo, 2001). The first narcotic unit was established in 1967; drug education in school was initiated by the police's youth section, which was established in 1971; and the first specialized drug treatment services were launched, the so-called 'Youth Stations' (*Nuorisoasemat*) (Kinnunen & Lehto, 1998). New drug legislation came into force in 1972 and heralded an era of very strict drug policy, which lasted until the end of the 1990s. The police became the central definer of drug problems (Hakkarainen, 1992; Kinnunen, 2008;Kainulainen, 2009;). Drug use practically vanished from the statistics in the 1970s, and the few remaining user groups were severely marginalized (Hakkarainen, 1992; Kinnunen & Lehto, 1998). The zeitgeist was clearly present in a substance treatment law enacted in 1986, which did not address drug problems in particular but discussed 'substance abuse problems' in general. Hakkarainen (1992) has referred to the 1980s as the period of 'stabilized development'. Although there was use and some experimentation among youths, this took place on a small scale and in criminalized circles.

The 'second drug wave' occurred in the latter part of the 1990s. The rapid increase in use of injections and associated individual and public health harms (HIV as well as hepatitis A, B, and C, and the peak in the drug-related deaths at the end of the 1990s) forced public officials to adopt new treatment and control measures and to rethink Finnish drug policy (Tammi, 2007). After fierce debates in parliament, the media, and between representatives of different ministries, harm reduction became a central policy option, leading to the launching of new treatment services, changes in social and healthcare legislation, and new ways of discussing drug problems and drug users at the beginning of the 2000s: 'injecting drug use', 'injecting drug users', and 'opioid dependency'. Medicine returned as the central area of expertise; for instance, with the appearance of 'best practice' treatment guidelines (Tammi, 2007). The first needle and syringe programme opened in 1997, and a few years later the first large-scale opioid maintenance treatment projects began (Perälä et al., 2013; Selin et al., 2013). However, restrictive drug policy measures were also strengthened (Kinnunen, 2008). All in all, the second drug wave had a lasting impact on the 'drug question' in Finland. The prevalence of drug use has remained at the same level as at the start of the wave. Current policies no longer aspire to a completely 'drug-free' Finland anymore but instead seek to minimize drug use's most significant harms and professional crime.

Generally, in Finland drugs have always represented an anomaly. During the most expansive period of the welfare state, in the 1970s and 1980s, drug use and users were mainly managed within a criminal framework and were not, for example, recognized as distinctive patients in need of specialized services. Over the course of the 1990s and 2000s, drug users' right to treatment became acknowledged in many ways, yet now, in the context of the so-called post-expansive welfare state, drug use is confronted by shrinking treatment budgets. Nowadays, drug use and drug problems are a permanent fixture of public policy discussions in Finland and have thus normalized to some extent (Hakkarainen et al., 2007).

3.2.3 **Sweden**

In the latter half of the 1800s and the first part of the 1900s, it was essentially medical doctors who formulated the drug problem in Sweden. These doctors witnessed negative side effects of drug consumption and dependency on various drugs that they had prescribed to their patients. The drug problem thus remained an individual problem handled by doctors themselves. The main aims were to avoid side effects and to cure drug use through medical expertise. The explanations for the problems were linked to the preparations' intrinsic effects and to characteristics of the patients themselves. These unacceptable ways of using drugs were often described as *missbruk* (abuse), but the urge to use drugs was also referred to as a disease of the will (Edman & Olsson, 2014).

Early-twentieth-century desires to tighten drug laws were never realized, and medical definitions of the drug problem were not significantly affected (Lindgren, 1993; Olsson, 1994). The transformation of drug use to a public and social problem began with the introduction of amphetamines and similar stimulants around the time of World War II. Based on very positive appreciations of the substances' medical properties among physicians, amphetamine use became popular, and over the next two decades use of the drug spread across large segments of the population. However, as amphetamines became an important part of the criminal subculture, moral connotations adhered to drug use, and it started being depicted as a threat to young people. As medical perceptions and disease concepts were ill-suited to understanding the phenomenon, the medical perceptions faded away, and legal and social explanations emerged.

Towards the mid-1960s, the drug problem reached such perceived proportions that governmental action was deemed necessary. In 1968, the drug issue was institutionalized via a drug policy programme. The key elements of this programme were measures against smuggling and selling drugs as well as drug treatment. The drug problem was formulated as a serious threat to society and to youths in particular. Actions against the manufacture, smuggling, and sale of drugs were assembled in a new law. Beds at various treatment centres were created, stimulated by government subsidies (Edman, 2012). Drug consumption was conceptually elaborated upon in the public report preceding the national drug policy of 1968: *narkotikamissbruk* (drug abuse) was defined as 'every non-medical use of narcotics', while *narkomani* (narcomania) was defined as 'an urgent need to keep abusing narcotics' (SOU 1967:25, p. 22). Drug addiction was described as pathological, and this 'disease' was often defined by some sort of dependency. However, this did little to clarify the situation, since the concept of dependency was—and remains—semantically obscure in Sweden. The distinction between drug abuse and narcomania was also deliberately blurred by the Swedish Minister of Health and Social Affairs in his ambition to avoid strict definitions in the government bill for coercive psychiatric treatment of drug users (Edman, 2009).

With the exception of coercive treatment measures in the 1970s, the drug problem remained primarily a social problem for most of the twentieth century. A contributing factor was the mismatch between drug users and the medical system. The population of users consisted predominantly of young, physically and mentally healthy criminals who used amphetamine. The description of drug use as a disease was therefore useless. In the twenty-first century, medical descriptions of the drug problem have been more frequent. A quest for evidence-based methods has made diagnostic manuals like the DSM-IV and ICD-10 more attractive; neurobiological and neuropsychological research has offered new explanations for drug consumption; and efforts to adopt an international vocabulary has, in some areas, replaced an older conceptual understanding of drug use with that of dependency or addiction (Edman & Blomqvist, 2011; Edman & Olsson, 2014). We thus currently experience the slightly contradictory conceptualization of a disease that is curable by severe repression: medicalized conceptions of drug consumption can coexist with criminalization not only of drug possession but also of the very practice of drug consumption.

To conclude this brief overview of drug policy history in Denmark, Finland, and Sweden as well as the evolving terminology in each country, it is evident that drug policies have developed quite differently in the three countries despite their common framework of the Nordic welfare state model. Though they share a historic common starting point in viewing drug-related problems as primarily social problems since the 1960s, the social problem approach has been interpreted very differently. The Finnish and Swedish welfare conceptions of drug use and drug users have tended to see these phenomena as alien to society. In

Denmark, drug problems are more based on a conceptualization of drug use and drug users as part of society and as a 'normal' social problem. In addition, the individual has been granted a more prominent position in Danish welfare policies, in contrast to the more collective responsibility approaches that can be identified in Finnish and Swedish policies and conceptions. These fundamental conceptions of the drug problem as a social problem seem to have played important roles in the constitution of the policy space within which the problem has been discussed. To further examine the similarities and differences between the countries, we continue by analyzing policy developments and conceptualizations of drug-related issues across three specific topics. Each topic has been contested and widely discussed in each country. They thus highlight the different ways each country conceptualizes and seeks to manage drug-related issues.

3.3 Three contested topics: sanctions, coercive treatment, and substitution treatment

3.3.1 Sanctions against drug users

In the framework of analyzing policy spaces and thereby how a country conceptualizes drug-related issues, a key question is the extent to which a country's drug policy criminalizes drug users, and how punishment is balanced with other types of interventions such as prevention and treatment (Benoit, 2003; Dorn, 1995). To examine this, we compare the legal provisions against drug users in Denmark, Finland, and Sweden. Although drug-related problems have primarily been constructed and conceptualized as social problems in all three countries since the 1960s, their drug control policies have developed differently. This is despite a convergence towards a rather punitive policy in recent years, led by Denmark's adoption of a more punitive policy in the early 2000s.

In Finland and Sweden, the long-lasting punitive policy conceptions of drug users were grounded in an ambition to create a drug-free society, as indicated in the historical overview. In Sweden, for instance, the Drug Criminal Law of 1968 criminalized all forms of drug handling. When the Drug Criminal Law was enacted, the maximum penalty for serious drug offences was four years' imprisonment, raised to six years in 1969 and to ten years in 1972. Increased penalties have been motivated by the changing and deteriorating drug situation, more widespread use, increase in serious crime, and increased internationalization. Träskman (2011, p. 62) describes the rapid increase in the maximum penalty as a 'Nordic carousel' in which Sweden, Norway, and Finland rapidly increased the maximum penalties relative to other countries.

Repressive drug control was strengthened at the expense of prevention and treatment during the 1980s. The criminalization of drug use in 1988 in Sweden (with a subsequent increase in penalties in 1993) is one of the more remarkable control policy initiatives. This and other drastic measures can be considered manifestations of an ideology aimed at creating a drug-free society, which has overshadowed other political visions (Träskman, 1995). This goal was first formulated by moralistic anti-drug organizations but soon taken over by the political establishment (Lenke & Olsson, 1999). Since the early 1980s, an important aspect of the model has been the doctrine that this goal will be realized primarily through actions against individual drug users.

Finland, too, has traditionally followed a restrictive drug policy (Kainulainen, 2009; Kinnunen, 2008; Hakkarainen, 1992). The Narcotics Act enacted in 1972 (42/1972) adopted a very restrictive approach to the use, sale, and trafficking of drugs, and enshrined the official vision of all drug-related activities as 'aggravated' crimes. One purpose of the legislation was to control drug experimentation among youths by signalling that all activities associated with drugs could lead to serious judicial consequences.

Drug legislation has, however, represented a paradox in Finnish criminal policy (Kinnunen, 2008). According to the principles of humanist and neoclassical criminal policy adopted in the early 1970s, Finnish criminal law is generally supposed to be used very sparingly, avoiding heavy sanctions. Furthermore, the legislator is usually reluctant to increase the authority of the police as this could lead to the erosion of citizens' privacy. Drug control has, however, been an exception. For instance, unlike other criminal activities, where sanctions became more moderate in the 1970s, the sanctioning of drugs and drug users was strengthened. It was considered 'natural' that drug users were handled by law-enforcement officials and not by social and healthcare professionals or public health authorities. Control has also often fallen upon the users even though the official aim has been to concentrate on professional crime and international drug trafficking. Police, prosecutors, and courts seldom use the possibility of waive sanctions against drug users (Kainulainen, 2009).

Unlike in Sweden and Finland, the aim of a drug-free society has never been articulated in Denmark. As mentioned in the overview, *possession* of illicit drugs for personal use was made a criminal offence in 1955, whereas *use of* illicit drugs is also criminalized in Finland (1992) and Sweden (1988). This legislation was introduced to control the drug scene that had developed during the 1940s. In the 1960s, young people started using cannabis and later opiates and LSD imported from abroad. To prevent a professional drug market, and inspired by similar legislation in Norway and Sweden (Asmussen & Jepsen, 2007), Denmark amended the Penal Code to give up to six years' imprisonment for violations of the legislation involving drug trafficking and dealing. However, as a condition for passing this legislation, a majority in parliament required that provisions were taken to ensure that the new legislation would not 'rub off' on drug users and criminalize young people experimenting with drugs, allowing offenders of this sort to instead be let off with a caution. This caused Danish drug policy to be bifurcated: criminal justice policy seeks to reduce drug supply; welfare policy seeks to reduce drug demand.

Drug use was seen as a consequence of rapid and fundamental sociocultural changes that had affected Danish society since the 1950s (Houborg, 2008). According to this view, 'the drug problem' was a product of society itself and should be addressed through the development of specific social policies.

Although there was a gradual narrowing of the lenient policy towards drug users, particularly during the 1990s and early 2000s, this two-tier thinking was the ideological basis for Danish drug policy until 2004. In that year, an amendment to the Law on Euphoriant Substances repealed the depenalization policy and instead introduced a zero-tolerance policy on all possession of illicit drugs. Drug use was no longer (or to a lesser extent) explained in social terms, and drug users were thus no longer seen as subjects of social government. Rather, in reports from the National Board of Health and in popular discourse, young people tended to be conceptualized as rational consumers of intoxicating substances, who did not distinguish between legal and illegal substances. In line with a neoconservative political rationality, punishment should thus give drug users an incentive not to use drugs and should function as general prevention (Houborg & Bjerge, 2011). The zero-tolerance policy made it possible to waive charges only in rare instances, such as for people who were dependent on drugs and who had very few economic means. This option is, however, rarely used (Houborg, 2014).

Generally, Danish policies have until recently been eager to conceptualize drug problems as 'normal' social problems, whereas the punitive policies of Sweden and Finland are mainly grounded in paternalistic policies. In this sense, the political rationalities that inform the relationship between state and drug user in the three countries may be seen to differ. In Denmark, more emphasis is placed on individual users as well as their rights and motivations, whereas Finland and Sweden have conceptualized drug use as something alien that requires prohibition and punishment by collective approaches.

3.3.2 **Coercive treatment**

Another much-debated topic in the Nordic countries has been whether to use coercion in treatment. Just as with the topic of sanctions on drug users, opinions regarding the use of coercion are closely related to how drug problems are conceptualized (Benoit, 2003; Dorn, 1995). Following Benoit, the history of socializing or individualizing risks of drug use as matters of collective or individual responsibility affects the extent to which drug policies emphasize control or welfare strategies. Denmark, Finland, and Sweden have a long history of involuntary treatment of people with alcohol problems, but coercive drug treatment is one area in which the countries' drug policies differ (Lehto, 1994)—thereby highlighting how differently drug use has been conceptualized.

Coercion is articulated as an important aspect of Swedish drug treatment, and it has been argued that the social problem description has been an important basis for this paternalistic treatment (Edman & Stenius, 2007; Kaukonen & Stenius, 2005). The first legislation regulating the coercive treatment of alcohol users came into force in 1916. The possibility of producing legislation to cover the treatment of substance use besides alcohol was occasionally discussed but never realized. When the drug problem made a more public appearance in the 1960s, new treatment programmes were established, but no specific drug treatment legislation was launched. The legislation on alcohol treatment, in which alcohol use was articulated as a social rather than a medical problem, was considered by many to be repressive, class-based legislation, and unsuitable as a model for drug treatment legislation. Instead, the need for coercion was linked to a diagnosis of the drug consumer as 'sick' (Edman & Stenius, 2014). The most tangible consequence was that coercive treatment of drug users was exclusively dealt with in psychiatric institutions during the years 1969–1981.

Criticism against coercive treatment of both alcohol and drug users grew during the 1970s, but coercive care of alcohol and drug users was based on two radically different problem descriptions. How could one conceptually understand measures against the socially troublesome alcohol abuser and sick drug user within the same legislation? After years of work, the right-of-centre minority government suggested that users of both alcohol and drugs should be subject to compulsory care within psychiatry. The government had to argue that not only drug users but also alcohol users were sick people in need of coercive psychiatric treatment. However, this met serious resistance from the council on legislation, the standing committee on social questions, and parliament. The conceptual framing of all drug problems as diseases was seen as a mistake, and coercive measures were to be examined by yet another investigation (Edman, 2009, 2011).

Consequently, the coercive treatment law of 1982 did not mention dependency or disease-like conditions. The aim was to motivate clients towards further voluntary care. The investigating committee took every measure to distance itself from medical-psychiatric descriptions of use. *Need for care* was the criterion for intervention, a need that resulted from regular consumption. Criteria for enrolment could be when the client put 'his physical or mental health in grave danger' or when he or she 'as a result of abuse was likely to come to seriously harm himself [or herself] or those nearest to him [or her]' (SFS, 1981:1243, § 3). There was no need to speculate upon disease-like conditions behind this behaviour. An attempted conceptual shift in the motivations for coercive treatment is evident in the Abuse Investigation from 2011, which took a highly medicalized view on drug treatment. It leaned on the DSM-IV and ICD-10 (Edman & Olsson, 2014). The investigation's proposals were, however, not realized. In January 2013, the government minister responsible decided to retain a more socially oriented description of the mechanisms of abuse (SoU, 2012/2013: 18).

Finland has never had distinct legislation or policies regarding the coercive treatment of drug users. Due to the restrictive and control-oriented nature of Finnish drug policy, treatment played, all in all, a minor role in the management of drug users until the 1990s. If coercive treatment methods were seen as necessary, drug users were treated under the same legislation as people suffering from alcohol problems. Until the beginning of 1970s, the typical context for treating drug users was mental health hospitals, and coercion took place under the auspices of mental health law. Since the mid-1980s, use of coercive methods has been quite rare, and treatment of drug users has highlighted the principles free will and client autonomy (Leppo, 2012).

Traditionally, the Finnish substance abuse treatment system has nevertheless been quite control-oriented in its principles and practices. The Finnish Alcoholic Act of 1936 brought with it the first specific institutions for people suffering from substance problems. 'Alcoholics', as they were referred to in the law, could be committed against their will on the grounds of endangering themselves or their environment or due to continual arrests for drunkenness. Although the institutions were considered treatment facilities, their purpose was to guide people towards a 'virtuous' and 'regular' life through hard physical and mental labour (Malinen, 2009). The institutions were only for men, and committal periods could last as long as four years. Substance-abusing women were treated in their own institutions. If they were believed to suffer from mental health problems, they were committed to mental hospitals. If there was 'indecency' involved, they were placed in vagrancy institutions under the auspices of the vagrancy law, but both men and women were treated mostly in mental health hospitals (Kinnunen & Lehto, 1998).

In 1962, new substance abuse treatment legislation adopted a slightly more lenient and therapeutic orientation towards substance abuse problems, but prevailing vagrancy law meant that coercion was still possible and widely used. For drug users, the significant context of treatment continued to be mental health hospitals, and there is some evidence that young people in particular were committed to these institutions against their will (Kinnunen & Lehto, 1998) In the mid-1970s social scientists and jurisprudents initiated the 'forced help' debate in public, which labelled existing treatment methods as demeaning and started to demand radical changes both in legislation and treatment practices. This prompted a significant decrease both in forced committals due to substance problems and in the duration of the committals. Many of the statutes that had previously allowed coercive methods were repealed, and citizens' legal protection was improved. The clearest turning point was the enactment of a new substance abuse treatment law in 1987, which overruled the old vagrancy law of the 1930s and adopted a quite 'client-centred' approach. This law is still in place today. The change in practices did not, however, concern drug users to the same extent as it did other substance users; according to the drug legislation of the 1970's they were conceptualized as criminals, rather than as people suffering from substance abuse problems and in need of treatment.

Current substance abuse treatment law makes it possible to use coercive methods in the handling of substance abuse problems in three instances: in cases of violent behaviour, in cases of risk of a serious health hazard or life-threatening situation caused by substance abuse (e.g. alcohol poisoning), and in cases of an underage individual Coercion is, however, seldom employed and the coercive sections of the law have generally been considered as a dead letter: still in principle in effect, but hardly ever used in practice. There have been, however, continuous efforts to change the legislation. In particular, the growth in substance use among women has created pressure to increase the compulsory treatment of women, with changes in Norwegian legislation serving as an example. The 'client' nevertheless retains many rights, and the principle of respecting 'client autonomy' continues to be very important (Leppo, 2012; Malinen, 2009).

Unlike in Finland and Sweden, the social problem description in Denmark was part of the basis for dismissing involuntary treatment (Houborg, 2008). Apart from the possibility of committing alcoholics who had committed criminal offences to institutions for 'drunkards', the use of coercion in treatment has historically been part of social welfare legislation. Until 1961, this legislation contained provisions that made it possible for social authorities to commit applicants for social benefits, or members of their household, to alcohol treatment as a condition for receiving benefits (Møller, 1945). Various special institutions existed for 'drunkards' but not for people with drug problems. The reasons are probably that until the 1940s, people with drug problems mainly came from the middle class, and drug treatment took place in psychiatric institutions. With regard to coercive commitment to psychiatric treatment, the 1938 legislation on hospitalization of mentally ill individuals made it possible to use coercion in treatment if patients were a danger to themselves or others, or if the possibility of curing the illness would be considerably less without hospitalization. The problem with drug users was that they could rarely be diagnosed as mentally ill, nor could they be said to be an immediate danger to themselves or others (Nimb, 1972).

The limited access to coercive treatment has often been problematized. The arguments for introducing coercive treatment have either been that lack of self-control makes it very difficult to treat people who are dependent on drugs or that people with drug problems are a danger to themselves or others (Behrendt et al., 1971; Møller, 1945). However, when the issue has been discussed, it has been dismissed—or considerably weakened—with references to civil rights. For instance, during the 1960s and 1970s, coercive treatment became a much-debated issue. The issue was not just about how to balance respect for drug users' civil rights against a curative ambition, but also about which conceptualization of drug dependency should form the basis for Danish drug policy. As mentioned earlier, a social understanding of 'drug abuse' as a meaningful socially learned behaviour came to dominate drug treatment in the 1960s and 1970s. The proponents of this conception were strongly opposed to coercive treatment for legal reasons and because they believed that coercion rested on a mistaken conception of the drug problem. They argued that just as each step of the way into drug abuse had been voluntary and meaningful for the drug user, so should each step of the way out of drug abuse through treatment also be voluntary and meaningful (Andersson, 1971; Ulff-Møller & Jørgensen, 1971). Coercion would counteract this. A 'principle of voluntary treatment' was thus articulated as the basis for drug treatment (Houborg, 2008; Kløvedal, 1970).

In 1992, new legislation on the possibility of coercively retaining drug users in treatment was enacted, but this was a very cautious form of involuntary treatment, which could best be conceptualized as 'voluntary involuntary treatment', resting on a principle of 'triple voluntariness' (Järvinen & Skretting, 1992). First, the regional council that was the political and administrative body in charge of drug treatment needed to decide whether to include this measure in its treatment policy. Second, the regional council needed to decide in each case whether to make a contract with the client concerning retention in treatment. Third, the contract was voluntary for the client, and the client could not be refused other treatment if he or she refused to make a contract. The measure has not had a great impact as it has only been used once.

Again, it does not seem that a 'social' conception of drug problems in a Nordic welfare state context necessarily leads to a paternalistically based coercive policy. One reason for the different emphases on involuntary treatment in the three countries could be that they balance paternalism and collective responsibility with individual autonomy and responsibility in different ways. Denmark has often placed greater emphasis on individual responsibility and less on collective responsibility and is closer to a liberal welfare regime in its political rationalities than are Finland and Sweden. Sweden continues to emphasize a very paternalistic approach, whereas some opening towards more focus on the individual's rights has recently been evident in Finland.

3.3.3 Substitution treatment

Substitution treatment is often highlighted as worthy of investigation in order to identify a country's drug policy space (Edman, 2012; Frank et al., 2013; Perälä et al. 2013). This has been a much-debated topic in all three countries, not least because of the problems of integrating medical treatment into a social conception of drug problems.

In Sweden, the reason for debating MMT can be traced to an increasing number of opiate users the 1970s (Johnson, 2003). MMT appeared to be a potential problem solver, but due in part to unsuccessful legal prescription attempts in the 1960s and a strong public conception of drug problems as a social problem, MMT was only used on a very small scale and was highly criticized until the mid-1980s (Skretting & Rosenqvist, 2010). However, the opinion swung, partly because of positive results from the small but effective MMT programme and partly because of the HIV/AIDS epidemic. For example, the organization Physicians Against AIDS (established in 1984) promoted the idea that drug abuse should be considered a disease to be treated within the healthcare system. In 1987, the National Board of Health and Welfare decided to increase the number of MMT places, a decision that marked the end of the most intense resistance to methadone.

Although MMT has been cautiously expanding since the 1990s, a certain hesitancy can be discerned (Johnson, 2007; Skretting & Rosenqvist, 2010). The development of MMT can in part be seen as an expression of a medicalization of drug treatment and drug policies, and an increased interest in evidence-based practices in social services (Johnson, 2007). The promotion of fear of HIV/AIDS as well as a successful MMT trial laid the groundwork for a conceptual shift in policy. Drug users were reconceptualized as patients with medical problems that required medical treatment, not as objects of social reform. From a comparative perspective, Swedish MMT must nonetheless be described as highly regulated and restrictive, and as part of Swedish drug policy, where treatment is designed to lead to total abstinence (Selin et al., 2015). Nevertheless, it is no longer debated whether MMT should be permitted; instead the debate is how treatment should be regulated and what demands should be placed on patients.

In the mid-1970s, an experimental MMT programme for people with chronic opiate addiction began in Finland's psychiatric medical care. The programme did not last long, and in the 1990s there were still only very few people receiving opioid substitution treatment (OST) (Holopainen, 1998). The official 'non-medical' approach to substance use treatment highlighted the important role of social workers and various socio-pedagogic methods, and the general impression was that there was no need for specific treatment facilities and approaches targeting drug use and drug users (Kinnunen & Lehto, 1998; Perälä et al., 2013).

A significant increase in opioid use at the turn of the millennium led to rapid changes in treatment policies and legislation. Substitution treatment slowly began proliferating (Kaukonen & Stenius, 2005), with several memoranda promoting medical and pharmaceutical treatment of opioid dependency t (Hakkarainen & Tigerstedt, 2002). At first, the criteria for enrolling in OST were quite strict. The first decree on OST, issued in 2003, stated that the goal of treatment was rehabilitation. Only people assessed as motivated for treatment and quitting drug use could enrol. This led to very long evaluation and waiting periods during the first years of OST, as well as to growing criticism of treatment practices, both from the treatment professionals promoting the treatment and from people suffering from opioid dependency (Perälä et al., 2013).

Since then, the entrance to treatment has, however, facilitated significantly. In 2005, OST became part of the "treatment guarantee law", giving clients the right to receive treatment within six months of seeking treatment. This significantly facilitated entrance to OST treatment. A new decree issued in 2008 made harm reduction OST possible, which lowered the threshold of the treatment even more.; Drug users in this programme were not required to stop using illicit drugs anymore, making OST possible also for those drug users, who still used for instance cannabis or amphetamine occasionally. Currently, OST has become a key pillar of Finnish drug policy (Selin et al., 2013), and, somewhat paradoxically, OST has turned in a very short period of time from being a controversial and heavily criticized treatment method to being virtually the only treatment option available for drug users. This has led to growing debate about and conceptualizations of the medicalization of Finnish substance use treatment as well as the lack of other treatment options (Perälä et al., 2013; Selin et al., 2013).

Until the 1970s, Danish drug users were primarily perceived as young people who required resocialization. However, a growing number of drug users could not fit into the treatment system. These drug users would sometimes ask GPs to prescribe methadone, which some GPs did. In this way a de facto two-pronged system developed: an official drug-free social treatment system alongside an unofficial medical treatment system (Houborg, 2013). In 1979, there was a small opening for the most severe cases to receive MMT after careful vetting, but it was not until the mid-1980s that MMT was accepted as a normal treatment modality. In 1984, graduated treatment goals were introduced in drug services to offer help, care, and treatment to particularly marginalized drug users, even when they were actively using illegal drugs. The introduction of such harm reduction strategies as part of Danish drug policy included the possibility of using MMT on a much larger scale; fear of the HIV/AIDS epidemic helped push the MMT agenda forward in Denmark (Frank et al., 2013). In the wake of this development, concepts of health *care* to improve people's quality of life rather than *cure* addiction became integral to the conceptualization of marginalized drug users.

Despite MMT's political acceptance, it was managed quite restrictively in the 1980s and 1990s because of ideological scepticism in the treatment system. As a consequence, many drug users still preferred MMT from GPs. In 1998, a change in medical legislation gave the public drug treatment system a monopoly on medical drug treatment. This led to a gradual shift in the culture surrounding MMT within the drug treatment system, with doctors and medical perspectives gaining significance (Frank et al., 2013). The increasing importance of the medical perspective was accompanied by an increasing articulation of somatic problems among drug users, problems resulting from an aging population of drug users. Currently, substitution treatment—including treatment with buprenorphine and heroin maintenance treatment—is the most frequently used treatment modality, and access to medical treatment has become a legal right for drug users. In other words, Denmark is currently experiencing an increased focus on medication and the management of drug-related issues as health-related problems; marginalized users in MMT are increasingly being conceptualized as palliative 'patients' rather than as citizens in need of rehabilitation (Andersen & Järvinen, 2007).

Altogether, Denmark, Finland, and Sweden are experiencing a turn towards medicalization as a means of managing and conceptualizing drug users as patients in substitution treatment. Nevertheless, the means of managing drug use from this perspective is quite different across countries. Again, Swedish policies echo the paternalistic approach that has been traced in the analysis of the previous topics, whereas Denmark seems to conceptualize a much more liberal approach. Finland can perhaps best be described as applying an approach between those of the two other countries, though shifting in a more liberal direction, not solely aiming for a drug-free society.

3.4 Conclusion

The Nordic welfare states are quite similar in many ways, so much so that many have referred to them as belonging to a 'Nordic welfare model' (Christiansen et al., 2005; Kvist et al., 2012). But when it comes to conceptualizing drug-related issues and policies, the differences between the countries are often so great that it is problematic to speak of *one* Nordic model, notwithstanding a certain convergence in recent years. One might say that the present-day drug policies of Denmark, Finland, and Sweden have a common basis in a conceptualization of 'the drug problem' as a *social* problem that should be managed primarily through social reform and various kinds of social expertise. It is thus characteristic that even though 'the drug problem' was initially constituted as a medical problem, medicine came to play a residual role in the understanding and management of drug problems. Recent years have, however, shown a tendency towards increased 'medicalization' of how the drug problem is conceptualized.

Despite these commonalities, there have been and still are significant differences between the three countries' drug policies. The main difference concerns the use of coercion and punishment directed at drug users, which in turn may be grounded in different ways of constructing the drug problem as a social problem. In both Finland and Sweden, the welfare approach to conceptualizing and managing drug problems was coupled with a conception of drug use and drug users as 'alien' to society. In Denmark, the welfare approach rested upon an understanding of drug use and drug users as part of society—as a 'normal' social problem. These fundamental conceptions of the drug problem as a social problem seem to have played an important role in constituting the policy space within which the problem has been discussed and measures to manage it have been constructed.

Furthermore, the main theoretical basis for constructing drug use as a social problem has differed among the countries. Whereas 'the principle of voluntariness' in Danish drug treatment rests upon a conception of social learning in which individual meaningfulness, choice, and responsibility play an important role, social treatment in Finland and Sweden seems to have been more closely linked to moral treatment. Central to understanding the policy space of each country is also the emphasis placed on individual as opposed to collective responsibility. It is thus significant that in Finland and Sweden, it has been possible to develop policies in which collective responsibility for cure or normalization of the individual has been more important than the autonomy of the individual to make his or her own choices. In Denmark, emphasis has been on the individual's autonomy and responsibility, and when provisions for involuntary treatment were established, they were highly ambivalent and have in fact almost never been used. When sanctions against drug users, coercive treatment, and substitution treatment are taken as a whole, Sweden represents the most paternalistic, conservative rationality towards the management of drug-related issues, followed by Finland, which also has a tradition for managing these issues rather strictly—a perspective that, at least with respect to substitution treatment, is currently softening. Despite its emphasis on a high level of collective responsibility, Denmark is more closely related to a liberal welfare regime than the other countries, because much more emphasis is generally placed on the individualization of risks of drug use.

There are, however, signs of convergence between the drug policies of the three Nordic countries. On the one hand, Denmark has moved towards the punitive policies of the other countries with respect to drug users, articulating a (neo) conservative law-and-order policy of a sort that has dominated the drug control policies of Sweden and Finland for many years. On the other hand, Finland has reduced emphasis on involuntary treatment, focusing instead on clients' rights, leaving Sweden to uphold the emphasis on coercion. Concerning substitution treatment, there is also convergence. This is mainly because substitution treatment has become more acceptable in Finland and Sweden, whereas Denmark has a long and extensive tradition of substitution treatment. In this sense, similar welfare systems conceptualize and exercise different policy spaces due to specific national developments, traditions, and actors influencing the drug policy agenda.

3.5 Acknowledgement

The chapter stems from a collaboration between Nordic researchers interested in developments within the addiction field. These researchers have been directly and indirectly involved in producing a special issue of *Nordic Alcohol and Drug Journal* (2014) on concepts and institutions for managing alcohol, drug, and tobacco problems in the Nordic countries from 1880 to 2010. Many of the researchers involved in this special issue are also involved in the EU-based *Addictions and Lifestyles in Contemporary Europe* (ALICE RAP) programme, which includes historical and contemporary analysis of the addiction fields in various European countries.

References

Andersen, D. & Järvinen, M. (2007). Harm Reduction – Ideals and Paradoxes. *Nordic Studies on Alcohol and Drugs*, **24**(3): 235–252

Andersson, J. (1971). Ungdomsklinikken. In E. Jepsen (Ed.), Afvigerbehandling. København: Thaning & Appels Forlag. 50–74.

Asmussen, V., & Jepsen, J. (2007). Dansk narkotika-kontrolpolitik—aktuelt og historisk. In J.S. Pedersen (Ed.), Ret og Samfund 2007, 109–136. København: Frydenlund.

Baldwin, P. (1990). The politics of social solidarity: class bases of the European welfare state 1875–1975. Cambridge: Cambridge University Press.

Behrendt, F.B., Jersild, M., Strömgren, E., Voigt, J., Dalgaard, J.B., Kjærsgård, H.H., & Sørensen, B.F. (1971). Forslag til bekæmpelse af narkoarttikamisbruget. *Ugeskrift for Læger*, **133**(27), 1330–1331.

Benoit, E. (2003). Not just a matter of criminal justice: states, institutions, and North American drug policy. *Sociological Forum*, **18**(2), 269–294.

Christiansen, N.F., Petersen, K., Edling, N., & Haave, P. (2005). The Nordic model of welfare: a historical reappraisal. København: Museum Tusculanum Press.

Dorn, N. (1995). A European analysis of drug enforcement. In G. Estievenart (Ed.), Policies and strategies to combat drugs in Europe. Florence: Martinus Nijhoff Publishers, 159–169.

Edman, J. (2009). What's in a name? alcohol and drug treatment and the politics of confusion. *Nordic Studies on Alcohol and Drugs*, **26**(4), 339–353.

Edman, J. (2011). En sjukdom? Narkotikamissbrukarna och den politiska diagnosen 1967–1981. In B. Olsson (Ed.), Narkotika. Om problem och politik. Stockholm: Norstedts Juridik, 139–159.

Edman, J. (2012). Swedish drug treatment and the political use of conceptual innovation 1882–1982. *Contemporary Drug Problems*, **39**(3), 551–566.

Edman, J. & Blomqvist, J. (2011). Jakten på den verksamma vården. Kunskapssträvanden och målsättningar inom den svenska missbrukarvården under ett sekel. In B. Olsson (Ed.), Narkotika. Om problem och politik. Stockholm: Norstedts Juridik, 101–13.

Edman, J., & Olsson, B. (2014). The Swedish drug problem: conceptual understanding and problem handling 1839–2011. *Nordic Studies on Alcohol and Drugs*, **31**(5–6), 503–526.

Edman, J., & Stenius, K. (2007). From sanatoriums to public injection rooms: actors, ideas and institutions in the Nordic treatment systems. In J. Edman & K. Stenius (Eds.), On the margins: Nordic alcohol and drug treatment 1885–2007. Helsinki: NAD. 339–361.

Edman, J., & Stenius, K. (2014). Conceptual carpentry as problem handling: the case of drugs and coercive treatment in social democratic welfare regimes. *International Journal of Drug Policy*, **25**(2), 320–328.

Esping-Andersen, G. (1990). The three worlds of welfare capitalism. Cambridge: Polity Press.

Frank, V. A., Bjerge, B., & Houborg, E. (2013). Shifts in opioid substitution treatment policy in Denmark from 2000–2011. *Substance Use & Misuse*, **48**, 997–1009.

Hakkarainen, P. (1992). Suomalainen huumekysymys [The Finnish drug question]. Helsinki: Alkoholitutkimussäätiö.

Hakkarainen, P. & Tigerstedt, C. (2002). Ristiriitojen huumepolitiikka—huumeongelman normalisaatio Suomessa [Contradicting drug policy—the normalization of drug policy in Finland.]. In M. Heikkilä & M. Kautto (Eds.), Suomalaisten hyvinvointi 2002 [Welfare in Finland 2002]. Jyväskylä: Stakes, 250–269.

Hakkarainen P., Tigerstedt, C., & Tammi, T. (2007). Dual-track drug policy: normalization of the drug problem in Finland. *Drugs: Education, Prevention and Policy*, **14**, 543–558.

Holopainen, A. (1998). Narkomaanin ja ammattiauttajan kohtaamisesta [On the encountering of the drug addict and the treatment worker]. In O. Kontula (Ed.), Huumeidenkäyttäjät Suomessa [Drug users in Finland]. Helsinki: Kirjayhtymä, 194–204.

Houborg, E. (2008). Youth, drugs and the welfare state. In V. Asmussen et al. (Eds.), Drug policy: history, theory and consequences. Aarhus: Aarhus University Press, 181–208.

Houborg, E. (2010). Control and welfare in Danish drug policy. *Journal of Drug Issues*, **40**(4), 783–804.

Houborg, E. (2013). Methadone a contested substance: Danish methadone policy in the 1970s. *International Journal of Drug Policy*, **24**(6), e73-e80.

Houborg, E. (2014). Construction and handling of drug problems in Denmark from the 1870s to the 1980s. *Nordic Studies on Alcohol and Drugs*, **31**(5–6), 527–550.

Houborg, E., & Bjerge, B. (2011). Drug policy, control and welfare. *Drugs: Education, Prevention and Policy*, **18**(1), 16–23.

Houborg, E., & Vammen, K.S. (2012). Hashbekymringer 1965–1969. In V.A. Frank & H.V. Dahl (Eds.), Cannabis—forbrug, interventioner og marked i Danmark. Aarhus: Aarhus University Press, 23–49.

Järvinen, M., & Skretting, A. (1992). Tvangsbehandling—symbolpolitik og paternalisme. In M. Järvinen & A. Skretting (Eds.), Missbruk och Tvångsvård, vol. 27. Helsingfors: Nordiska nämnden för alkohol-och drogforskning (NAD). 171–181.

Jepsen, J. (2008). Danish drug control policy 1945–2007. In V. Asmussen et al. (Eds.), Drug policy: history, theory and consequences. Aarhus: Aarhus University Press. 151–180.

Johnson, B. (2003). Policyspridning som översättning. Den politiska översättningen av metadonbehandling och husläkare i Sverige. Lund: Statvetenskapliga institutionen.

Johnson, B. (2007). After the storm; developments in maintenance treatment policy and practice in Sweden 1987–2006. In J. Edman & K. Stenius (Eds.), On the margins: Nordic alcohol and drug treatment 1885–2007. Helsinki: NAD. 259–287.

Kainulainen, H. (2009). Huumeidenkäyttäjien rikosoikeudellinen kontrolli [Criminal control of drug users]. Helsinki: Oikeuspoliittisen tutkimuslaitoksen julkaisuja. 245.

Kaukonen, O., & Stenius, K. (2005). Universalism under re-construction: from administrative coercion to professional subordination of substance misusers. In N. Kildal & S. Kuhnle (Eds.), Normative foundation of the welfare state: the Nordic experience. New York: Routledge, 130–148.

Kinnunen, A. (2008). Kriminaalipolitiikan paradoksi. Tutkimuksia huumausainerikollisuudesta ja sen kontrollista Suomessa [The paradox of criminal policy: studies of drug crime and its control in Finland]. Helsinki: Oikeuspoliittisen tutkimuslaitoksen julkaisuja. 233, 59–68.

Kinnunen, A., & Lehto, J. (1998). Drug treatment at the margins. In G. Hunt & H. Klingemann (Eds.), Drug treatment systems in an international perspective. Thousand Oaks, CA: Sage, 48–61.

Kløvedal, M. (1970). Frivillighedsprincippet i praksis. *Mentalhygiejne*, **23**, 212–215.

Kvist, J., Fritzell, J., Hvinden, B., & Kangas, O. (2012). Changing social equality; the Nordic welfare model in the 21st century. Bristol: The Policy Press.

Lehto, J. (1994). Involuntary treatment of people with substance related problems in the Nordic countries. In M. Järvinen & A. Skretting (Eds.), Missbruk och Tvångsvård, v. 27. Helsingfors: Nordiska nämnden för alkohol-och drogforskning (NAD). 7–32.

Lenke, L., & Olsson, B. (1999). Swedish drug policy in perspective. In J. Derks et al. (Eds.), Current and future drug policy studies in Europe: problems and research methods. Freiburg: Ed. iuscrim, Max-Planck Institute für Ausländisches und Internat, 135–166.

Leppo, A. (2012). Precarious pregnancies: alcohol, drugs and the regulation of risks. Helsinki: Sosiaalitieteiden laitoksen julkaisuja. 3, 57–61.

Lindgren, S-Å. (1993). Den hotfulla njutningen. Att etablera drogbruk som samhällsproblem 1890–1970. Stockholm/Stehag: Symposion Graduale.

Malinen, A. (2009). Inte har vi tvingat dig dit? Synen på tvången och autonomi i social-och misbrukarvården hos myndigheter och klienter i dagens Finland. In K. Stenius & L. Johansson (Eds.), Socialt medborgarskap och lokal missbrukavård. En studie av missbrukarvården i Lahtis, Kotka, Tavastehus, Norrköping, Västerås och Växjö från 1930-talet till 2000-talet. Stockholm: SoRAD–Forkningsrapport nr. 55, 250–269.

Møller, K.O. (ed.). (1945). Stimulanser. København: Gyldendal.

Nimb, M. (1972). Misbrug af euforiserende stoffer i Danmark i 1950'erne med efterundersøgelse i 1972. København: Københavns Universitet.

Oksanen, A. (2008). Kenraalit vauhdissa ja sotilaat sammuksissa: sotaa huumeissa ja humalassa [Drugs and addictions during the Second World War in Finland]. In S. Näre & J. Kirves (Eds.), Ruma sota: Talvi-ja jatkosodan vaiettu historia [The ugly war: the silent history of the Second World War]. Helsinki: WSOY 181–205.

Olsson, B. (1994). Narkotikaproblemets bakgrund. Användning av och uppfattningar om narkotika inom svensk medicin 1839–1965. Stockholm: CAN.

Partanen, J. (2002). Huumeet maailmalla ja Suomessa [Drugs in Finland and in the other countries]. In O. Kaukonen & P. Hakkarainen (Eds.), Huumeidenkäyttäjä hyvinvointivaltiossa. [The drug user in the welfare state]. Helsinki: Gaudeamus, 13–37.

Perälä, R., Hellman, M., & Leppo, A. (2013). Behind the scenes: the justifications for opioid maintenance treatment in Finland. *Substance Use & Misuse*, **48**(11), 954–965.

Pontoppidan, K. (1883). Den kroniske morfinisme. København: Th. Linds Boghandel.

Rose, N. (1999). Powers of freedom—reforming political thought. Cambridge: Cambridge University Press.

Salasuo, M. (2001). Mihin pilvi katosi? Huumeaallon taittuminen 1970-luvulla [Where did grass disappear? the subsiding of the first drug wave in the 1970s]. In T. Onnela (Ed.), Pyhä huumesota. Huumepolitiikan pelkoja ja utopioita [Holy drug war: the fears and utopians of drug policy]. Helsinki: Vihreä Sivistysliitto, 192–198.

Selin, J., Perälä, R., Stenius, K., Partanen, A., Rosenqvist, P., & Alho, H. (2015). Opioid substitution treatment in Finland and other Nordic countries: Established treatment, varying practices. *Nordic Studies on Alcohol and Drugs*, **32**(3), 311–324.

Selin, J., Hakkarainen, P., Partanen, A., Tammi, T., & Tigerstedt, C. (2013). From political controversy to a technical problem? fifteen years of opioid substitution treatment in Finland. *International Journal of Drug Policy*, **24**, e66–e72.

SFS. (1981). Lag om vård av missbrukare i vissa fall. 1243.

Skretting, A. & Rosenqvist, P. (2010). Shifting focus in substitution treatment in the Nordic countries. *Nordic Studies on Alcohol and Drugs*, **27**(6), 581–597.

SoU. (2012/2013: 18). God kvalitet och ökad tillgänglighet inom missbruks-och beroendevården.

Storgaard, L.L. (2000). Konstruktionen af dansk narkotikakontrolpolitik siden 1965. København: Jurist-og økonomforlagets Forlag.

SOU. (1967: 25). Narkotikaproblemet. Del 1: Kartläggning och vård. no. 25.

Tammi, T. (2007). Two-tracks drug policy: normalization of the drug problem in Finland. *Drugs: Education, Prevention & Policy*, **14**(6), 543–558.

Träskman, P. O. (1995). Drakens ägg—den narkotikarelaterade brottskontrollen. In D. Victor et al. (Eds.), Varning för straff. Om vådan av den nyttiga straffrätten. Stockholm: Fritze.

Träskman, P. O. (2011). Narkotikabrotten och kontrollen av bruket av narkotika genom straffrättsliga medel. In B. Olsson (Ed.), Narkotika. Om problem och politik. Stockholm: Norstedts Juridik, 43–72.

Ulff-Møller, B., & Jørgensen, F. (1971). To modeller for udvikling af stobrug blandt skoleelever i Danmark. *Socialt Tidsskrift*, **47**(1–2), 427–438.

Chapter 4

WHO expert committees and key concepts for drugs, alcohol, and tobacco, 1949–2013

Suzanne Taylor, Virginia Berridge, and Alex Mold

4.1 Introduction to the WHO expert committees and key concepts for drugs, alcohol, and tobacco

While other historical chapters of this book have studied national and regional situations, this chapter provides an international perspective by examining the role of the World Health Organization (WHO) and its expert committees in disseminating concepts around addiction in relation to illicit drugs, alcohol, and tobacco from 1949 to 2013. Three time periods are surveyed: 1949–1963, when intense discussion of concepts and terminology in relation to drugs and alcohol occurred and the substances were discussed as separate issues; 1964–1989, when the concept of dependence emerged, ushering in the potential for a combined approach to the substances, and also when discussion of tobacco arose; and the 1990s onwards, when a more sustained combined approach to the substances developed and the WHO exercised its constitutional powers to establish an international convention on tobacco. Major questions considered in this chapter include:

- What were the concepts discussed in relation to illicit drugs, alcohol, and tobacco?
- What terms were used and how were they defined?
- What were the similarities and differences in terminology across the substances?
- How were the expert committees situated within the WHO, and where did responsibility lie for each substance?
- What was the impact of the professional composition of committees?
- How did the terminology used in expert committee reports compare to that of the International Classification of Diseases (ICD), the standard diagnostic tool for epidemiology, health management and clinical purposes and conventions?

Review of the WHO expert committees demonstrates considerable engagement with concepts and terminology, and the importance of the WHO in establishing and shifting the conceptual boundaries between these substances. It highlights increasing linkages between the three substances under consideration; a more combined approach to research and treatment, but differences in control; early involvement with the problems of substance use and earlier discussion of tobacco than has generally been indicated in the existing literature; and the problems involved in the creation of standardized definitions at the international level. Box 4.1 provides a list of acronyms pertinent to this chapter.

Box 4.1 Key acronyms used in relation to the WHO expert committees and key concepts for drugs, alcohol, and tobacco, 1949–2013

ADS: Alcohol-Dependence Syndrome
ARD: Alcohol-Related Disability
ECAPD: Expert Committee on Addiction-Producing Drugs
ECDD: Expert Committee on Drug Dependence
ECDLPA: Expert Committee on Drugs Liable to Produce Addiction
ECDPD: Expert Committee on Dependence-Producing Drugs
FCTC: Framework Convention on Tobacco Control
ICD: International Classification of Diseases
PSA: Programme on Substance Abuse
SACTob: Scientific Advisory Committee on Tobacco Product Regulation
TFI: Tobacco Free Initiative
TobReg: WHO Study Group on Tobacco Product Regulation
UN: United Nations
WHA: World Health Assembly
WHO: World Health Organization

4.2 Historiography: role of the WHO, expert committees, and concepts and terminology around addiction in relation to drugs, alcohol, and tobacco

A literature review was carried out on secondary material on the WHO and illicit drugs, alcohol, and tobacco. This included topics on the history of the WHO, the development of international control mechanisms, WHO expert committees, and other relevant mechanisms such as the ICD and UN Conventions. Much literature on the WHO has concentrated on its role in combatting infectious diseases. Health promotion and public health has also been discussed and since the 1970s there has been interest in international substance control of illicit drugs and alcohol. The mechanism of the expert committee has been examined demonstrating its importance in the development of concepts, terminology, and definitions. Bruun et al. (1975) examined expert committees on drugs and alcohol and highlighted their significance in the development of key concepts; the importance of a committee's composition, policy imperatives, and outputs. Room (1981) has written extensively on this topic, focusing on alcohol and drugs. His analysis demonstrated the fluctuating focus of committees and major turning points, such as the 1992 ECDD (Room, 1997). Room uncovered significant shifts in terminology; for example, the transition from 'habit' and 'addiction' to 'dependence', and from 'alcoholism' to 'alcohol-related problems' (Room, 2005; Room & Babor, 2005; Selvaggio, 1984). He also considered the development of alcohol and drug categories in instruments such as the ICD, revealing its relationship with the WHO, problems of cross-cultural applicability of terms such as 'dependence', differentials between lay and technical understandings, and cross-drug applicability of terms (Room, 1984, 1997, 1998).

Edwards (2007), reviewing the WHO's 1977 report on alcohol-related disabilities, highlighted the lack of commonly accepted terminology as an obstacle to research and policy. His work emphasized the shift to 'disability' as the preferred term to describe the social burden resulting from disease. The changes in the WHO structure—for example, the Programme on Substance Abuse (PSA) which sought to bring a combined approach to substance abuse in the 1990s—have also attracted commentary (Babor, 2003; Grant, 1993). Work has largely considered these substances separately.

Tobacco has not been considered in relation to drugs and alcohol. Little has been said about expert committee discussion of tobacco despite its inclusion in WHO discussions from 1970. The Framework Convention on Tobacco Control (FCTC) in 2005 is noteworthy. Taylor and Bettcher (2000) analyzed the development of international health law. Collin et al. (2002) discussed the FCTC in the context of accelerating globalization. Civil society contributions to the negotiation process proved important for tobacco (Mamudu & Glant, 2009); Yach and Bettcher (2000) demonstrated that the tobacco industry increasingly attempted to influence agencies such as the WHO. Likewise Weishaar et al. (2012) have pointed to the transnational tobacco corporations' efforts to undermine the FCTC. The applicability of the framework to other substances has been the focus of a number of works (Jernigan et al., 2000; Lien & Deland, 2011;

Room & Babor, 2005). A final aspect of the literature is that it is generally written by non-historians, many employed or connected to the WHO. Although this has the advantage of insider knowledge, it tends to lack context and to be allied to an activist perspective (Moser, 1980; Yach & Monteiro, 2011; see also the conversations with Mackay, 2013; Moser, 1984; and Room, 2012).

The existing literature has demonstrated the importance of expert committees, but it has largely reviewed the substances individually and tends to concentrate on drugs and alcohol, not tobacco. Tobacco has been studied but with a greater focus on the development of the FCTC rather than its longer history at the WHO. As noted, the literature has largely been written by those with connections to the WHO rather than by historians. In this chapter we consider the three substances together under the umbrella of 'concepts of addiction'. We examine the relationship between concepts and terminology across these three substances, and extend their consideration from the involvement of the WHO in 1949 through 2013.

4.3 **Methodology: the WHO expert committees, Technical Report Series, and WHO archives**

As well as the literature review summarized earlier, the research examined printed reports and archival material. Examination of original printed material focused upon the *Technical Report Series*, which published findings of the expert committees; reports on illicit drugs, alcohol, and tobacco were reviewed. Other primary material included WHO Conventions, texts of which were surveyed for pertinent terms. Terms used in the ICD in relation to drugs, alcohol, and tobacco were reviewed. Although rarely utilized, we surveyed material held in the WHO archives in Geneva. Unfortunately, the archive does not hold minutes of meetings, but it does hold other relevant documentation, such as correspondence between committee members.

4.4 **WHO expert committees on illicit drugs and alcohol, and the early development of terminology, 1949–1963**

WHO expert committees are the highest official advisory bodies to the Director-General of WHO and member states. They are established by the WHO World Health Assembly (WHA) and each committee makes recommendations on a subject of interest to the WHO. Members are chosen from WHO expert advisory panels, temporary advisers, representatives from international organizations, nongovernmental organizations, and professional associations. The ECDD has been one of the most active committees, meeting every two years since it was established in 1949 (undergoing various title alterations). It has played a central role in the international drug control system, making recommendations to the United Nations Commission on Narcotic Drugs on control measures. In contrast, alcohol and tobacco committees, not needing to make scheduling decisions in relation to international conventions, have met less frequently, often in response to a WHA resolution calling for research on a particular area of emerging interest.

This chapter splits the expert committee discussions into three time periods: 1949–1963, when intense discussion of concepts and terminology in relation to drugs and alcohol occurred, and the substances were discussed as separate issues; 1964–1989, when the concept of 'dependence' emerged and ushered in the potential for a combined approach to the substances, and when discussion of tobacco arose; and the 1990s onwards, when a more sustained combined approach to the substances developed, and the WHO exercised its constitutional powers to establish an international convention on tobacco.

Between 1949 and 1963, terminology was a crucial factor in discussions (see Table 4.1). In relation to illicit drugs, the main term used was 'habit-forming'; the first committee established in 1949 was named the Expert Committee on Habit-Forming Drugs. Members were pharmacologists/chemists, and discussions centred on the status of various substances in relation to the conventions on controlled drugs (WHO, 1949).

But attention turned to a new term—'addiction'—and in 1950 the committee was renamed the Expert Committee on Drugs Liable to Produce Addiction (ECDLPA). Attempts were made to differentiate between the two terms. A 'habit-forming' drug was described as 'one which is, or may be, taken repeatedly without the production of all of the characteristics outlined in the definition of addiction and which is not generally considered to be detrimental to the individual and to society' (p. 7). The term referred mainly to 'psychic dependence', whereas 'drug addiction'—which implied both 'psychic' and 'physical' dependence—was preferred by the committee. Addiction was defined as 'a state of periodic or chronic intoxication, detrimental to the individual and the society, produced by the repeated consumption of a drug (natural or synthetic) . . . a psychic (psychological) and sometimes a physical dependence on the effects of the drug'. (p. 7) 'Dependence,' a term that would become prominent in the 1960s, was mentioned but not defined. The committee decided that 'habit-forming' should be eliminated from all texts, and urged governments to consider medical research on 'drug addiction'.

Table 4.1 Major WHO expert committee reports, 1949–1963

Date	Committee	Output	Substance	Major shifts in terminology
1949	Expert Committee on Habit-Forming Drugs	[First report]	Drugs	Habit-forming; habituation
1950	Expert Committee on Drugs Liable to Produce Addiction	Second report	Drugs	Addiction
1951	Expert Committee on Mental Health: Alcoholism Subcommittee	First report	Alcohol	Alcoholism; chronic alcoholism; addictive drinking
1952a	Expert Committee on Drugs Liable to Produce Addiction	Third report	Drugs	
1952b	Expert Committee on Mental Health Alcoholism Subcommittee	Second report	Alcohol	Alcoholism; excessive drinkers
1954a	Expert Committee on Alcohol	First report	Alcohol	Alcohol intermediate between habit-forming and addiction-producing
1955a	Expert Committee on Alcohol and Alcoholism	'Alcohol and Alcoholism: Report of an Expert Committee'	Alcohol	Excessive drinking rather than alcoholism; problems of alcohol use or problem use, of which alcoholism is one aspect
1956	Expert Committee on Drugs Liable to Produce Addiction	Sixth report [of a meeting held in Geneva, 24–29 October 1955]	Drugs	
1957	Expert Committee on Addiction-Producing Drugs	Seventh report	Drugs	Addiction-producing drugs
1958	Expert Committee on Addiction-Producing Drugs	Eighth report	Drugs	Interest in treatment for the 'addict'
1959	Expert Committee on Addiction-Producing Drugs	Ninth report	Drugs	
1960	Expert Committee on Addiction-Producing Drugs	Tenth report	Drugs	
1961	Expert Committee on Addiction-Producing Drugs	Eleventh report	Drugs	Medical control of addicts
1961	Convention	UN Single Convention on Narcotic Drugs	Drugs	

The distinction between the two was important because attempts were made to link these concepts to control measures. A 1952 committee acknowledged that the term 'addiction' implied a serious state, one which 'must be rigidly controlled.' In contrast, drugs resulting in 'habituation' were thought more innocuous, as they 'cause no sociological damage and do not need rigid control' (WHO, 1952a, p. 10). This split proved problematic because some 'borderline' drugs such as alcohol fell into an intermediate position and were outside international control.

Discussion of alcohol focused more on the condition of 'alcoholism', taking a more medical approach. The first expert committee, the WHO Expert Committee on Mental Health's Alcoholism Subcommittee of 1951, focused on conceptual discussion of 'alcoholism' (WHO, 1951). Its membership, mainly psychiatrists, was chaired by Dr G.A.R. Lundquist, assistant professor of psychiatry at Langbro Hospital, Stockholm. The secretariat included Prof. E.M. Jellinek, a WHO consultant on alcohol and dean of the Yale Institute of Alcohol Studies; much of the historical literature has focused on his work on alcoholism. The subcommittee made clear that 'alcoholism' was a disease and a social problem in which public health services should play a significant role in prevention and treatment.

Terminology occupied a large part of the committee's report. The initial term used was 'chronic alcoholism', but this was quickly discredited due to cross-cultural misunderstandings—an important consideration for the WHO working in a global environment. 'Alcoholism', defined as 'any form of drinking which in its extent goes beyond the traditional and customary dietary use or the ordinary compliance with social drinking customs,' was seen to have a more consistent meaning and became the preferred term. 'Alcoholism' was refined into stages which were important because of their clinical significance and potential treatment regimes. In referring to 'addictive drinking', the subcommittee noted the work of the 1950 Expert Committee on Drugs Liable to Produce Addiction (ECDLPA) on definitions for 'addiction'. The subcommittee acknowledged similarities to drugs of addiction, but maintained a distinction in that it was 'uncertain whether or not the pharmacological concomitants of drug addiction exist . . . creating a physical dependence on the drug.' This led to pressure for a new subcommittee under the ECDLPA to examine the potential 'drug of addiction', alcohol, rather than the 'disease' of 'alcoholism'.

The Subcommittee on Alcoholism met again in 1951. Chaired by Dr M. Schmidt, chief psychiatrist, Department of Police, Denmark, it concentrated on practical and specific aspects of 'alcoholism'. The previous subcommittee's provisional definition of 'alcoholism' was adopted for 'excessive drinkers', while alcoholics were defined as

> excessive drinkers whose dependence upon alcohol . . . shows a noticeable mental disturbance or an interference with their bodily and mental health, their inter-personal relations and their smooth social and economic functions. . . . They therefore require treatment. (WHO, 1952b, p. 10–16)

The position of alcohol in relation to other drugs became increasingly important, especially as the term 'addiction' became dominant in relation to illicit drugs. An Expert Committee on Alcohol was created and reported in 1954 (WHO, 1954). The composition of the alcohol committee differed from that of the previous committees on 'alcoholism'; it comprised mainly pharmacologists and physiologists (later committees also had a wider range of disciplines). The committee was chaired by Dr Lundsgaard, professor of physiology at the University of Copenhagen, and included professors of pharmacology such as Dr L. Goldberg from Stockholm and Dr J. Mardones from Santiago, Chile, an associate professor of medicine from Stanford University, and L.D. MacLeod from the Burden Neurological Institute, Bristol. They discussed broader ramifications—etiological, epidemiological, sociological, and anthropological—as opposed to purely pharmacological or clinical concerns.

The committee drew on the work of the 1950 ECDLPA, which added to the confusion, because alcohol and 'alcoholism' could not easily be fitted into the definition of 'drug addiction'. Alcohol was placed in a category of its own, one intermediate between 'addiction-producing' and 'habit-forming'. Concepts pertaining to the pharmacological position of alcohol remained unclear; for instance, the term 'tolerance to alcohol' was seen as causing misunderstandings. A distinction was deemed necessary between 'tolerance' related to addiction-producing drugs of the morphine type and 'tolerance' associated with alcohol. 'Withdrawal symptoms' also proved contentious, as in the alcohol field, the term 'withdrawal symptoms' was used, whereas the term 'abstinence syndrome' was used in the case of drug addiction of the morphine type. Thus the committee was unable to match the definitions between alcohol and illicit drug terminology. The separate category for alcohol was necessitated by the difficulty of drawing a line between the presence and absence of addiction-producing properties (WHO, 1954). The subcommittee pressed for a further meeting incorporating both clinicians and experimental workers to attempt further clarification.

This borderline position of alcohol remained important for the Expert Committee on Alcohol and Alcoholism which met in 1955 (WHO, 1955). Jellinek and Wolff had left; a changing membership drew together pharmacologists, physiologists, psychiatrists, and members from both the Advisory Panel on Mental Health and the ECDLPA. Its mandate was to clarify basic concepts related to alcohol and the features of the problem in different countries. The committee reiterated the importance of 'alcoholism' as a medical problem in order to involve public health services. However, this was proving difficult due to inadequately defined terminology.

The introduction of the concept of 'problems of alcohol' or 'problem use' forced a broader consideration of the problem. This shift away from 'alcoholism' was important because it was 'excessive drinking' rather than 'alcoholism' which was a major problem for most countries. One approach was to cease using the term 'craving' and adopt 'physical dependence'. Though the 1955 committee acknowledged recent evidence which indicated a closer resemblance between responses to the withdrawal of alcohol and opiates, it concluded that there was no justification for a change in the position on alcohol. Instead, the preferred concept became the 'problems of alcohol', of which 'alcoholism' was just one aspect.

'Addiction' continued to pose problems for illicit drugs, and the renamed Expert Committee on Addiction-Producing Drugs (ECAPD) revisited the issue (WHO, 1957). Its membership began to broaden. Significantly, the committee included Dr L. Goldberg, who sat on the 1954 Expert Committee on Alcohol, and for the first time included a psychiatrist, Dr Pernambuco Filho, University of Rio, Brazil. The distinction between 'addiction' and 'habit-forming' remained problematic. The committee was forced to refine the previous definitions, as follows:

> Drug addiction: Its characteristics include: (1) an overpowering desire or need or compulsion to continue to take the drug; . . . (2) a tendency to increase the dose; (3) a psychic (psychological) and generally a physical dependence on the effects of the drug; (4) detrimental effects on the individual and on society.
>
> Drug habitation (habit): (1) a desire (but not a compulsion) to continue taking the drug for the sense of improved well-being which it engenders; (2) little or no tendency to increase the dose; (3) some degree of psychic dependence on the effect of the drug but absence of physical dependence and hence of an abstinence. (p. 9–10)

These new definitions were to find some acceptance by the time of the 1960 committee but they were far from perfect. The committee complained that heterogeneous criteria had been included to meet the requirements of international control, but this made definitions difficult to interpret. Hence they reiterated the basis of control, which was related to risk to the community: the 'fundamental criterion for control is the extent to which these drugs induce behaviour disturbance and risk to the community' (WHO, 1960).

A significant shift appeared when interest expanded to the user and the methods of prevention and treatment as opposed to the pharmacological action of drugs. The issue of the 'addict' and 'treatment' appeared in the 1958 expert committee report (WHO, 1958) after pressure by the UN Economic and Social Council. It became significant as the committee pressed for an opportunity to comment on drafts of the 1961 UN Single Convention on Narcotic Drugs. The convention enshrined the term 'addiction', a term the expert committees would later try to replace. In 1959 the committee had raised disquiet over the schedules for the convention, the scope of control, and the treatment of drug addicts (WHO, 1959). Attitudes towards drug addicts and their treatment came to the fore in 1961 when the committee discussed the medical control of addicts. Though proposals for civil commitment of an addict (in the case of mental patients) to a medical panel were approved, they were not deemed a replacement for legal penalties (WHO, 1961). The 1962 committee pointed out that although 'withdrawal' must be the first step in treatment, for a 'cure' to be successful, 'rehabilitation' was necessary, and hence there was an immediate need for treatment and rehabilitation facilities.

In sum, during this period both drug and alcohol committees were active. Tobacco was not considered at this point. Drugs and alcohol were considered by separate committees, but concepts and terms were important areas of discussion for both committees. Drug committees initially were made up mostly of pharmacologists, but later were slightly widened to include other disciplines, notably the occasional inclusion of a psychiatrist and one member who had also sat on the alcohol committee. This period saw a shift from the term 'habit-forming' to 'addiction', though the term remained problematic. Drug committees had been established to provide advice in relation to pre-existing international drug control treaties, so the focus was on the substance, though there was a slight shift to consider the problems of use—for example, consideration of the 'addict' by the end of this period.

In contrast, there were no international treaties for alcohol control. Hence the WHO began with health concerns over the condition, not the 'drug'. Committees on alcoholism began as largely psychiatric-based and focused on the condition 'chronic drinking' and later 'alcoholism'. Later committees, which included pharmacologists, physiologists, and psychiatrists, considered 'alcohol' and the 'problems of alcohol use' and 'excessive drinking' rather than just 'alcoholism'. Although some similarities were drawn with illicit drugs, significantly, alcohol was deemed to occupy an intermediate position. Furthermore, in contrast with drug committees, alcohol committees began with an interest in prevention and rehabilitation and an acknowledgement of the significance of cultural differences in alcohol use.

4.5 The rise of 'dependence', tobacco, and the prevention of problems associated with substance use, 1964–1989

During the period 1964–1989, the concept of 'dependence' developed and opened the way for a combined approach to the substances. Though the 1971 UN Psychotropic Drugs Convention led to a focus on scheduling requirements rather than drug terminology and interest in alcohol declined by the 1980s, some influential reports emerged. These reports emphasized the concept of a medical rather than a penal approach, the threat to the community as well as the individual, and the need for prevention of both drug and alcohol 'related problems' rather than a narrow focus on supply. Additionally, during this period tobacco entered the WHO's consciousness as a serious global public health threat (Table 4.2).

Table 4.2 Major WHO expert committees reports, 1964–1989

Date	Committee	Output	Substance	Major shifts in terminology
1964	Expert Committee on Addiction-Producing Drugs	Twelfth report	Drugs	Dependence; drug abuse
1965	Expert Committee on Dependence-Producing Drugs	Fourteenth report	Drugs	Dependence-producing drugs
1966	Expert Committee on Dependence-Producing Drugs	Fifteenth report	Drugs	
1967	Expert Committee on Mental Health	Fourteenth report [of a meeting held in Geneva, 4–10 October 1966]	Alcohol and drugs	
1969	Expert Committee on Drug Dependence	Sixteenth report	Drugs	
1970	Expert Committee on Drug Dependence	Eighteenth report	Drugs	Psychotropic drugs and the qualifying term 'dependence-producing'
1970		C.M. Fletcher and D. Horn, 'Smoking and Health'	Tobacco	Less hazardous smoking/cigarette
1973	Expert Committee on Drug Dependence	Nineteenth report	Drugs	
1974	Expert Committee on Drug Dependence	Twentieth report	Drugs, alcohol, and tobacco	Problems associated with the use of psychoactive, dependence-producing drugs; includes alcohol and tobacco but tobacco excluded from pre-review

(continued)

Table 4.2 (continued) Major WHO expert committees reports, 1964–1989

Date	Committee	Output	Substance	Major shifts in terminology
1975	Expert Committee on Smoking and its Effects on Health	Smoking and its Effects on Health Meeting: Report	Tobacco	Psychic dependence and withdrawal; smoking habit; dependence adopted in relation to nicotine; involuntary exposure to smoke
1979	Expert Committee on Smoking Control	'Controlling the Smoking Epidemic'	Tobacco	Elimination; rejection of the safe cigarette
1980	Expert Committee on Problems Related to Alcohol Consumption.	Meeting (1979) in Geneva	Alcohol	Alcohol-related disabilities; alcohol dependence syndrome Problems related to alcohol consumption
1983	Expert Committee, Smoking Control Strategies in Developing Countries	Report	Tobacco	
1985	Expert Committee on Drug Dependence	Twenty-second report	Drugs	
1987	Expert Committee on Drug Dependence	Twenty-third report	Drugs	
1988	Expert Committee on Drug Dependence	Twenty-fourth report	Drugs	
1989	Expert Committee on Drug Dependence	Twenty-fifth report	Drugs	
1989	Expert Committee on Drug Dependence	Twenty-sixth report	Drugs	

A significant moment was the adoption of the term 'dependence' by the 1964 ECAPD, chaired by Dr N.B. Eddy, a pharmacologist and consultant on narcotics, National Institutes of Health, USA. The committee consisted largely of pharmacologists but did include one psychiatrist, Dr P. Kielholz, University of Basel, Switzerland. Moreover, the committee had a different emphasis: it welcomed the fact that other agencies, such as the Commission on Narcotic Drugs, were pushing for an increased emphasis on the sociological and economic aspects of 'drug abuse'. With the increasing number of drugs available and continuing confusion over 'addiction' and 'habituation', it had proved difficult to find a term that could be applied generally to 'drug abuse'. The concept of 'dependence' was seen as a common factor between the many varieties of drugs. Though the term had been loosely used previously, it became the preferred term, defined as

> a state arising from repeated administration of a drug on a periodic or continuous basis. Its characteristics will vary with the agent involved and this must be made clear by designating a particular type of drug dependence in each specific case. (WHO, 1964, p. 9)

Specific types of drug dependence were elucidated; for example, drug dependence of the morphine type. Crucially, 'dependence' was not linked to any type of control. The 1965 committee was renamed the Expert Committee on Dependence-Producing Drugs (ECDPD) (WHO, 1965).

But 'dependence' had flaws. Criticisms were made of the vagueness of the term, cross-cultural applicability, and cross-drug applicability. Furthermore, it created conflicts with the ICD. The section which covered drug addiction in the ICD contained a diverse list of terms, which the committee argued were not necessarily addiction-producing drugs in a pharmacological or legal sense. The report therefore recommended that 'drug dependence' be taken into account by the ICD.

There was added pressure for clarity when the committee's mandate was broadened in 1966 and again in 1969: from the determination of the control status of drugs to other aspects of 'drug dependence' and 'abuse' (WHO, 1969). The committee's name was also altered to Expert Committee on Drug Dependence (ECDD) in 1969. In addition to pharmacologists, membership of the ECDD was widened to include Dr A. Wikler, professor of psychiatry and pharmacology, University of Kentucky, and Dr P.H. Connell, a psychiatrist at the Bethlem and Maudsley Hospital, London. This shifting membership resulted in a shift towards the condition rather than a strict focus on the drug. 'Drug abuse' was defined as 'persistent or sporadic excessive drug use inconsistent with . . . acceptable medical practice.' 'Drug abuse' was deemed convenient on the grounds that there was no universally accepted term. By 1975 the term 'abuse' would be dropped by the WHO due to its stigmatizing connotations (Kramer & Cameron, 1975), though it remained in the ICD until 1992.

These developments meant that the split between alcohol and illicit drugs was harder to sustain. The WHO wanted to encourage authorities to look at 'alcohol and alcoholism and use and abuse of drugs together'. Although a more combined approach had been sought by the Expert Committee on Mental Health, this was more in relation to research (and to a lesser extent with treatment and education), as opposed to control measures (WHO, 1967b).

The increasingly combined approach to drugs and alcohol was reflected in the 1967 Expert Committee on Mental Health Services for the Prevention and Treatment of Dependence on Alcohol and Other Drugs (WHO, 1967a). This committee was chaired by Dr K. Evang, Director-General, Health Services of Norway, and consisted of sociologists, psychiatrists, neuropsychiatrists, and a pharmacologist. It also included representatives from the UN narcotic drug organizations, such as Mr A. Lande, secretary to the Permanent Central Narcotics Board, as well as those from the alcohol field, including Mr H.D. Archibald, director of the Alcoholism and Drug Addiction Research Foundation, Toronto, Canada. The broader disciplinary backgrounds reflected the committee's mandate, which was to consider the establishment of services for the prevention and treatment of 'dependence' on both alcohol and other drugs.

The rationale to combine the approaches was persuasive. The concept of 'dependence' brought the concepts around the differing substances closer together. The committee noted the similarities in causation and treatment, and the fact that drugs were themselves often used in combination. Research from the alcoholism field was also viewed as relevant to controlled drugs, and it was accepted that, although attitudes towards 'alcoholism' had shifted towards the therapeutic, this had not happened to the same extent with controlled drugs.

Tobacco, when it surfaced as an issue for the WHO, did so within a different framework: public health. A 1970 report of the Director-General (Fletcher and Horn, 1970), based on the work of Charles Fletcher and Daniel Horn (1970), leading anti-smoking campaigners, sought to establish the problem as worthy of consideration by the WHO by referring to the links to diseases such as lung cancer, as well as the increasing uptake of smoking, especially by women. The report led the WHO to affirm the hazards of smoking and to ban smoking in its own meetings. The concept of 'less hazardous smoking' arose, alluding to the development of 'less hazardous' cigarettes and methods of smoking. Other methods such as filters were also considered, and the report called for research on the effects on health of modifications in the constituents of cigarettes (WHO, 1970). A follow-up report in 1971 focused on potential methods of control (WHO, 1971). Legislation was considered important; for example, in enacting measures to encourage smokers to stop. The 'less hazardous cigarette' remained an option and differential taxation favouring the use of 'less harmful cigarettes' was discussed. Any economic losses from reduced tobacco revenue were expected to be offset by a healthier population. By the early 1970s, tobacco would enter discussions of the drug committees.

But the major focus of the early 1970s was psychotropic drugs, culminating in the UN Convention on Psychotropic Substances in 1971. Psychotropic drugs had become a priority for the committee in 1970, when draft protocols of the convention were sent to the ECDD. At this time the committee consisted mainly of pharmacologists, although there were two psychiatrists, one of whom was Dr M. Shepherd, Institute of Psychiatry, London. The convention necessitated refinement of the terminology. A link to 'dependence' was one criterion for control. The term 'psychotropic' applied only to substances specifically listed in one of the first four schedules; the committee accepted that many psychotropic substances used in medicine did not produce 'dependence'. Therefore, to avoid confusion, a qualifying term, 'dependence-producing', was introduced to be added when speaking of psychotropic substances to be controlled in the draft protocol. This committee also broached the concept of a medical rather than penal approach, emphasizing treatment and rehabilitation within public health services.

The 1973 committee reflected the rise of the public health population approach; it consisted of a wider range of disciplines, with epidemiologists and sociologists joining the pharmacologists and psychiatrists. This led to further refinements around the concept of 'dependence' with a focus upon 'dependence-producing drugs and more interest in the problems surrounding the use of such drugs' (WHO, 1973). 'Dependence' in itself was not necessarily considered harmful—in a broad sense, it could include tea and coffee—whereas drugs, such as alcohol, cannabis, and opiates, resulted in individual, public health, and social problems.

Thus by 1974 there was a shift in focus to prevention of the problems associated with drug use. The committee was chaired by Dr B.S. Brown, Director of the National Institute of Mental Health, Department of Health, Education, and Welfare, USA, and included several members of the UN Division on Narcotic Drugs, including Dr O.J. Braenden, and members of the International Council on Alcohol and Addiction. Dr H. Halbach, a professor of pharmacology at the University of Munich, was invited to consider what was known about preventing problems associated with the use of psychoactive, dependence-producing drugs. This shift meant that alcohol gained a higher profile because it was deemed more of a problem than many illicit drugs. Tobacco—the most widespread form of drug dependence—was also drawn into discussion. However, tobacco was excluded from pre-review (the preliminary stage to decide whether a substance should undergo a fully documented or critical review which might lead to the scheduling of a psychoactive substance) on the grounds that its psychotoxic effects were slight compared to other drugs (WHO, 1974).

Yet tobacco warranted its own expert committee (WHO, 1970). Following a 1974 resolution requesting that an expert group be convened, the Expert Committee on Smoking and its Effects on Health was created. It met in 1975 to summarize evidence on the harmful effects of smoking and to propose actions to discourage smoking. Hence, tobacco was isolated from committees concerned with illicit drugs; smoking entered the expert committee's realm from a public health perspective. This was reflected in its membership, which was mainly social medicine and public health experts, cardiologists, and policymakers (WHO, 1975b). It was chaired by Sir George Godber, the UK Chief Medical Officer, with Dr Sujoy B. Roy, professor and head of Department of Cardiology at the All-India Institute of Medical Sciences, New Delhi, acting as the person appointed by the committee to report on the proceedings of its meetings. Its members included Dr F. Beske, professor of social medicine and public health, Secretary of State, Ministry of Social Affairs, Kiel, Germany. Charles Fletcher acted as a temporary adviser. This committee reviewed the state of knowledge since Fletcher and Horn's 1970 report and reviewed the gamut of potential control measures, including warning notices, prohibition in certain public places, and protection of the rights of 'non-smokers', as well as quality control and education. Some terms used were similar to those adopted for alcohol and drugs, including 'psychic dependence' and 'withdrawal'. Although drug terminology had moved away from 'habit' or 'habitation' early on, the phrase 'smoking habit' was widely used in reports. Few terms were defined. In relation to nicotine, the term 'dependence' was adopted: 'Chronic use of nicotine produced[s] dependence and that for some people the disturbing nicotine withdrawal syndrome . . . contributes to the difficulty of giving up.' (p. 15) Thus the issue of 'withdrawal', developed in drug and alcohol committees, was picked up for tobacco, but differences were also identified: social reinforcement and 'dependence' were thought to develop faster with tobacco than with other drugs such as alcohol.

At the same time, the effects of smoking were accepted as extending beyond the individual user. What would become known later as 'passive smoking' was discussed as 'involuntary exposure to smoke.' The report noted potential damage to non-smokers: 'the non-smoker exposed to the side stream and mainstream of smokers in enclosed, ill-ventilated spaces such as cars and small offices may be exposed to harmful concentrations of smoke.' (p. 16) This threat to the wider community boosted the need for stricter control measures. Furthermore, by protecting the non-smoker it was hoped to reduce opportunities for smoking.

Threat to the wider community was an important concept for all these substances. This was especially true with alcohol. As discussed by Room (1984), work during this time focused on alcohol's impact on the community beyond the individual drinker. The question of 'alcohol disabilities' was discussed by a WHO Steering Group between 1973 and 1975, resulting in a broader focus than the 'alcoholic'. 'Alcohol-related disabilities' and later 'alcohol-related problems' became the focus at the WHO. The emphasis on 'disability' rather than disease was intended to draw attention to the need to reduce the consequences on the family and society, as well as the individual. Although concrete definitions were not deemed possible, a loose definition was the following:

> Alcohol-Related Disability is deemed to exist when there is impairment in the physical, mental or social functioning of an individual of some nature that it may be reasonably inferred that it is part of the causal nexus determining that disability. (Edwards et al. 1977)

By 1976 'dependence' was adopted by the alcohol field. Alcohol-dependence syndrome was seen as one variety of alcohol-related disability (ARD) and was adopted by the 1980 committee. Not all those with ARD were seen as alcohol-dependent but were at more risk of becoming so. 'Alcohol dependence' entered the ninth revision of the ICD.

Whereas with alcohol attempts were made to 'manage' associated problems, with tobacco the goal was elimination. Tighter control of the smoking epidemic was the primary focus of the 1979 tobacco expert committee. Membership was weighted to anti-smoking advocates. The committee was chaired by Sir George Godber, with Dr Nigel Grey, of the Anti-Cancer Council of Victoria, Australia, as rapporteur. Others included Dr K. Bjartveit, Chairman of the National Council on Smoking and Health, Oslo, and Dr L. Ramstrom, Director-General of the National Smoking and Health Association, Stockholm. Significantly, the aim was elimination, 'removal of the hazard not marginal reduction' (WHO, 1979). This meant that the concept of the 'safe cigarette' was rejected. Instead, potential methods of control leading to elimination were promoted, including control of advertising, health warnings, taxation, restrictions on smoking in public places, and evaluation of legislation. Crucially, this report marked the first calls for the use of WHO's constitutional powers to develop an international treaty.

To summarize, although the 1971 Psychotropic Convention came into force during this period and there was less discussion of concepts around illicit drugs as the committees became more involved in technical discussion over scheduling, there were significant developments. There were major changes to the drug committees' composition, with pharmacologists being joined by epidemiologists, sociologists, and those working in the alcohol field. There was also a shift in how the problems were conceptualized. 'Addiction' was replaced by 'dependence' and 'dependence-producing drugs', a move which brought potential for a more combined approach to the substances. As such, alcohol became an issue as it could be seen as a 'dependence-producing drug'.

Another important change was a shift in interest to not just the prevention of drug use but the limitation of problems once drug use had occurred. There were limited reports on alcohol, but, significantly, concepts developed around 'alcohol-related disabilities' and 'alcohol-related harm'. Importantly, smoking emerged as a public health problem and warranted the establishment of its own expert committee. Membership of the committee was broad both in geographical location and disciplines but with a medical/public health emphasis. The focus was on the elimination of smoking, though the idea of the 'less hazardous cigarette' emerged, and calls began for WHO to exercise its constitutional powers for an international legal approach to tobacco control.

4.6 A combined approach? the Programme on Substance Abuse and the Framework Convention on Tobacco Control, 1990–2013

The period from 1990 to 2013 is characterized by a more sustained combined approach to substance use. This was reflected in changes to the WHO structure, with the creation of the Division of Mental Health and the Prevention of Substance Abuse's Programme on Substance Abuse (PSA). This period is also marked by the development of global strategies for tobacco control, most notably the Framework Convention on Tobacco Control, which represented the first time the WHO had exercised its constitutional powers (Table 4.3).

Mounting pressure for a combined approach to drugs and alcohol was built into the structure of the WHO in the 1990s. The WHO's global strategy of 'health for all by the year 2000' led in 1990 to the creation of a new programme, the PSA, designed to prevent and control alcohol and drug abuse. This resulted in alcohol and drugs being briefly separated from the mental health division. Expert committees began to review the substances together. The Expert Committee on Health Promotion in the Workplace reviewed approaches to health promotion as a means of preventing both alcohol and drug problems. Alcohol and drug-related problems were defined as being applicable to any of the adverse accompaniments of drinking or drug-taking, and they could be related to either an individual drinker or to society (WHO, 1993b).

Table 4.3 Major WHO expert committee reports, 1990–2013

Date	Committee	Output	Substance	Major shifts in terminology/focus
1991	Expert Committee on Drug Dependence	Twenty-seventh report	Drugs	
1993a	Expert Committee on Drug Dependence	Twenty-eighth report	Drugs	Harmful use to replace abuse; dependence; disabilities or problems related to drug use of which 'dependence' was just one factor; alcohol consumption and levels of use; e.g. less heavy patterns of use; harm minimization
1993b	Expert Committee on Health Promotion in the Workplace	'Alcohol and Drug Abuse'	Drugs and Alcohol	
1995a	Expert Committee on Drug Dependence	Twenty-ninth report	Drugs	Different legal approaches to control but similarities of treatment options for drugs, alcohol, and tobacco
1999a	Expert Committee on Drug Dependence	Thirty-first report	Drugs	Tobacco included for pre-review
2000	Expert Committee on Drug Dependence		Drugs	
2001	Expert Committee on Drug Dependence	Thirty-second report		
2003a	Expert Committee on Drug Dependence	Thirty-third report	Drugs	
2006	Expert Committee on Drug Dependence	Thirty-fourth report	Drugs	

(*continued*)

Table 4.3 (continued) Major WHO expert committee reports, 1990–2013

Date	Committee	Output	Substance	Major shifts in terminology/focus
2006	Study Group on Tobacco Product Regulation	Meeting in Kobe, Japan, 28–30 June Scientific basis of tobacco product regulation	Tobacco	Attractiveness; harm reduction; dependence used as a synonym for addiction
2006	Expert Committee on Problems Related to Alcohol Consumption	[First report]	Alcohol	
2007a	Expert Committee on Problems Related to Alcohol Consumption	Second report	Alcohol	Alcohol-related harm; problems related to alcohol consumption; risk of harm; intoxication

The 1993 ECDD also considered alcohol, and—although it was initially outside of the PSA's remit—tobacco was also included in discussions. Membership was broad, including psychopharmocologists, addiction psychiatrists, epidemiologists, and policymakers. The director-general of the WHO had requested the committee look at strategies for reducing substance use and its harmful consequences. Crucially, the tenth edition of the ICD (ICD-10) included alcohol and tobacco in the list of psychoactive drugs with potential to cause mental and behavioural disorders, including 'dependence'. The committee discussed the concept of drawing together illicit and licit substances and coordinating their control mechanisms. In terms of tobacco, the committee argued that the 'dependence-producing' properties of nicotine and the severe health consequence of tobacco and nicotine warranted its inclusion in their discussions, thereby further expanding the committee's mandate.

In redefining the role of the committee, concepts and terminology occupied an important place. Many of the terms from the previous reports remained valid, but with new research findings there were important subtle shifts. 'Harmful use'—'a pattern of psychoactive drug use that causes damage to health, either mental or physical. . . . Harmful use of drugs by an individual often has adverse effects on the drug user's family, the community and society'—replaced the term 'abuse', which was deemed ambiguous (WHO, 1993a, p. 6). However, it was recognized that the term 'drug abuse' had entered numerous national laws and international conventions, so 'abuse' remained in operation.

'Dependence' remained dominant. The committee decided to follow the ICD-10 diagnostic guidelines and not make a distinction between 'physical dependence' and 'psychic dependence' in order to avoid clinical misunderstandings (WHO, 1993a, p. 5). However, there was a shift towards 'problems' or 'disabilities related to drug use', of which 'dependence' was just one. Further review of the term 'dependence-producing drug' drew nicotine and tobacco into consideration. The level of dosage of a drug now also came into prominence: 'A state of dependence is not necessarily harmful in itself, but it may lead to self-administration of the drug at dosage levels that produce deleterious physical or behavioural changes constituting public health and social problems' (WHO, 1993a, p. 6).

Research had led to a reconceptualization of alcohol consumption levels as a continuum and to an understanding that alcohol-related problems were related to consumption patterns. This was now seen as applicable to all substances, resulting in a change in focus towards those with 'less heavy patterns of use' (WHO, 1993a, p. 4). Thus concepts and terminology around levels of consumption were becoming important.

Discussion of 'harm minimization', 'harm reduction', or the 'preventing of problems associated with the use of psychoactive dependence-producing drugs' now explicitly appeared in texts; the committee highlighted the value of harm reduction as opposed to its potential for encouraging drug use (WHO, 1993a, p. 3).

Common approaches were brought together when another reorganization took place in 1995. At that time the Programme on Substance Abuse was amalgamated with the Division of Mental Health to create the Division of Mental Health and Prevention of Substance Abuse (WHO, 1997). Significantly, this division was involved with all psychoactive substances, licit or illicit, including tobacco, alcohol, and illicit drugs.

The 1995 ECDD reflected these changes, acknowledging that although different legal approaches existed for drugs, alcohol, and tobacco, there were significant similarities in treatment options. Consequently, the committee sought treatments that could be used across the three substances. Treatment and rehabilitation were meant to include 'comprehensive identification, assistance, healthcare, and social integration.' Consistent with growing interest in 'human rights' in relation to controlled drugs, inherent in the definition was the idea that all users should be treated 'with humanity and respect' (WHO, 1995a).

In 2000, the Department of Substance Abuse was merged with the Department of Mental Health to create the Department of Mental Health and Substance Abuse, under the Non-Communicable Disease and Mental Health cluster, thus bringing together common approaches to the management of mental health and substance use disorders. Amendments were seen as essential given the adverse attitudes towards drug users; the committee pressed for an update to the WHO (1994) *Lexicon of Alcohol and Drug Terms*, a tool for clinicians, administrators, and researchers, which had been established in 1994.

Tobacco had proved awkward for the ECDD. Although approaches to research and treatment had drawn substances closer together, approaches to control took a different track. The existing conventions were not deemed appropriate for regulating tobacco, because the only option would be prohibition, which was not viable. The idea of an alternative global mechanism for tobacco control was formalized in 1995 at the World Health Assembly (WHO, 1995b). By 1997 the PSA had a section specifically for tobacco—Tobacco or Health—and the development of an international framework was an important element of its strategy. It published *Guidelines for Controlling and Monitoring the Tobacco Epidemic*, advocating long-term, comprehensive tobacco control policies (WHO, 1998).

In 1998, after Gro Harlem Brundtland, a physician herself, became director-general of the WHO, tobacco control activities were set within a new structure. The Tobacco Free Initiative (TFI), run by Dr Derek Yach, aimed to raise the profile of tobacco control. Its role was to initiate a process to develop a framework convention that would permit member states to adopt a comprehensive tobacco control policy dealing with aspects of tobacco control that transcended national boundaries. While tobacco had been rejected for pre-review in 1996 by the ECDD, by 1999 this decision was reversed because of new evidence of greater liability for abuse (WHO, 1999a). In 2000, the WHO Framework Convention on Tobacco Control (FCTC) was adopted by the WHA, becoming the first international treaty negotiated under the auspices of the WHO (2003b); it came into force in 2005.

Terms such as 'addiction', 'nicotine addiction', 'addictive nature', and 'tobacco dependence' and 'cessation', were used but they were not defined in the treaty. 'Habit', while frequently adopted in discussions, did not appear in the treaty text. Definitions related more to the needs of the treaty, and so were focused more on issues of control, trade, and products than on usage. The definition of tobacco control included supply, demand, and 'harm reduction' strategies. 'Harm reduction' itself was not defined; the emphasis remained on elimination.

Engagement with definitions emerged via a new body. The Scientific Advisory Committee on Tobacco Product Regulation (SACTob) was established in 2000 with the objective to advise WHO on the most effective, evidence-based means to fill regulatory gaps in tobacco control and thus achieve a coordinated regulatory framework. In 2003 this advisory committee was formulized into a study group, and it became known as the WHO Study Group on Tobacco Product Regulation (TobReg). Its report of 2006–2008 considered product regulation, including cigarette contents. 'Dependence' was used as a synonym for 'addiction'; beginning in 2012, the term 'addiction' was dropped. Reflecting a focus on the consumer, the term 'attractiveness' crept in, a phrase that did not appear for drugs or alcohol. Reports noted that cigarettes were exempt from health and safety standards; the aim of the WHO FCTC was to lay the ground for future regulation of contents. Whereas the concept of a 'safe cigarette' had earlier been rejected, 'harm reduction' methods were again a feature. A detailed explanation of 'harm reduction' based on other organizations' definitions was provided, but the study group pointed out that any such action 'must not undermine prevention, cessation and reduction of exposure to second-hand smoke and, ideally, should support them' (WHO, 2007b).

The approach to alcohol followed that taken for tobacco rather than for 'illicit' drugs. The coordinated global public health approach became a feature of alcohol policy, which focused on reducing the problems of consumption. In 2001, Gro Harlem Brundtland spoke publicly on alcohol issues for the first time, and a WHO Alcohol Policy Strategic Advisory Committee was established. A WHO resolution in 2005 called for evidence-based strategies to reduce alcohol-related harm (WHO, 2005). The 2007 WHO Expert Committee on Problems Related to Alcohol Consumption pressed the WHO to develop a global action plan to reduce the harmful effects of consumption. The committee argued for clear definitions of alcohol-related terms, particularly in the area of policy.

Definitions reflected this altered focus; for example 'alcohol-related harm' and 'problems related to alcohol consumption' were seen as equivalent terms encompassing a wide variety of health and social problems at the individual and societal level (WHO, 2007a). Although 'harmful use' was in the ICD-10, the WHO expert committee argued for a broader understanding, one related to the public health aims of the WHO, in which the 'risk of harm' now appeared as a part of 'alcohol-related harm'. Distinctions, however, were drawn, and problems with the term 'harm reduction' in relation to alcohol noted (WHO, 2007a).

At the same time, the term 'intoxication' was introduced. Intoxication was defined as 'a predictable consequence of the ingestion of substantial quantities of alcoholic beverages in a limited period of time.' Although 'intoxication' was part of the ICD, the committee pointed out a number of factors that affected it, including cultural differences and the amount consumed. Intoxication was seen as leading to 'risk taking behaviours' such as unprotected sexual activity, which could lead to 'disabilities' and impose burdens on health services and third parties.

'Dependence' was again accepted with respect to alcohol. Significantly, the committee noted that if alcohol had been considered under the 1971 convention, it would have qualified for scheduling, as it constituted a public health and social problem (WHO, 2007a). However, as with tobacco, it was not considered practical to include alcohol in current conventions. Instead, by 2008 the WHO had drafted a global strategy which included national actions, such as policies for drunk driving, while at the international level priority areas included public health advocacy and partnership, as well as the production and dissemination of knowledge (WHO, 2010).

In sum, this period is characterized by a more sustained combined approach to substance use and its related problems. With drugs, in particular, prevention of drug use-related problems—of which 'dependence' was just one aspect—became important. In so doing, concepts of 'harm reduction/minimization' entered discussions. Common approaches, especially for treatment and rehabilitation, were examined, but differences in control policy remained. This is highlighted by the major development in the tobacco field with creation of the FCTC. Alcohol policy was reinvigorated with a focus on 'alcohol-related harm' and pressure for a global policy in light of developments in tobacco control.

4.7 **Conclusion: the development and role of the WHO expert committees in 'concepts of addiction' for drugs, alcohol, and tobacco**

This review of the WHO expert committees on illicit drugs, alcohol, and tobacco reveals attempts at the difficult task of standardization of terms around 'concepts of addiction', the development of an increasingly combined approach to these substances, moves to bring tobacco and alcohol into a public health agenda over which the WHO has control, and attempts to influence the illicit drug agenda.

WHO expert committees were very active in changing concepts and definitions around 'addiction'. The term 'habit-forming', and its replacement, 'addiction,' quickly proved unsatisfactory, especially in light of their links to control measures, as well as 'borderline' substances which could not be defined by either term. 'Addiction' was replaced by the concept of 'dependence' and a focus on 'dependence-producing drugs'.

The shift to 'dependence' highlighted similarities between illicit and licit substances. For example, alcohol became an issue, as it could be seen as a 'dependence-producing drug'. This opened the door to a more combined approach to the substances, at least in relation to research and treatment, although less so for control. A major change was a shift in interest not only to prevention of substance use but the limitation of problems or 'disabilities' once such use had occurred. Further refinement led to concepts around levels of consumption; for example, an increasing concern with 'excessive drinking' rather than a focus on 'alcoholism'.

A term that appeared in discussions for all these substances—although it proved contentious—was 'harm reduction'. This was interesting in the case of tobacco, for which there was emphasis on the concept of 'elimination'. However, even though elimination was impractical, concern remained for those unwilling or unable to quit; thus the concept of 'harm reduction' had to be considered. The balance between 'harm reduction' and 'elimination' proved difficult, as evidenced by the issue of 'less hazardous' or 'safer' cigarettes. Recently, it has led to much debate over e-cigarettes. Finally, although tobacco discussions largely drew on terms already established for alcohol and drugs, they also brought new terms such as 'consumer attractiveness' into the discussion.

Changing scientific disciplines within the committee system have played an important role in the development of concepts and terms. Early drug committees dominated by pharmacologists focused on the substance, whereas alcohol committees, initially dominated by psychiatrists, concentrated on the medical condition. Broadening the professional disciplinary base to include pharmacologists, psychiatrists, sociologists, and clinicians, and cross-fertilization between the committees, led to greater interest in treatment and rehabilitation and eventually in combined approaches. In contrast, tobacco committees had a medical/public health composition and focus from the start.

The organizational structure of the WHO has also been important. Alcohol and drugs were both placed under mental health but were initially considered by separate committees. Increasingly, however, linkages brought research and potential treatment options closer together. Nevertheless, approaches to control have differed. Control was a given for illicit drugs, with international mechanisms and conventions established within a penal framework developed prior to the creation of the WHO. But this was not the case for alcohol and tobacco. Alcohol committees increasingly sought to emphasize the medical aspects of the problem to ensure a public health–oriented approach. In contrast, tobacco, seen as an epidemic, even pandemic, entered WHO's consciousness as a public health issue, and one with added impetus due to the threat to the non-smoker. Tobacco's position in relation to the other substances is interesting. Initially considered separately, it was later incorporated into the PSA. Later still it began to follow its own track, leading to the formation of the FCTC whereby the WHO set the precedent for a convention under its own auspices. Alcohol became the only one of the three substances without some form of international control mechanism. WHO began to press for alcohol to be dealt with as a global public health issue and drew inspiration from the tobacco convention.

WHO committees did not operate in isolation. Differences existed between committees, conventions, diagnostic tools, and common usage of terms. In addition, there were time lags between committee discussions and changes to diagnostic mechanisms such as the ICD. For example, the WHO committees pressed the ICD to include 'dependence'. The committees might also be at odds with other organizations such as the American Psychiatric Association, which wanted to reinstate 'addiction' in the 2006 edition of its *Diagnostic and Statistical Manual*. While the ICD-11 has retained 'dependence', the psychiatric association proposed to replace it with 'substance use disorder'.

Finally, terminology is not fixed. Rather, it is in constant flux, due to changing scientific understanding, evolving drugs, and new delivery methods. Ever-changing policy imperatives, cultural differences, and attempting to meet the needs of different actors contribute to the mix. Thus the debates are ongoing around dosage, 'intoxication', and levels of use. The current debate concerning 'heavy use over time' as a replacement for the concepts discussed in relation to addiction (Rehm, 2013) suggests that the WHO and its expert committees will continue to play an important role.

References

Babor, T.F. (2003). Alcohol: no ordinary commodity: research and policy. Oxford: Oxford University Press.

Bruun, K., Pan, L., & Rexed, I. (1975). The gentlemen's club: international control of drugs and alcohol. Chicago: University of Chicago Press.

Collin, J., Lee, K., & Bissell, K. (2002). The Framework Convention on Tobacco Control: the politics of global health governance. *Third World Quarterly*, **23**, 265–282.

Cueto, T.M., & Fee, E. (2006). The World Health Organization and the transition from 'international' to 'global' public health. *American Journal of Public Health*, **96**, 62–72.

Edwards, G. (2007). How the 1977 World Health Organization report on alcohol-related disabilities came to be written: a provisional analysis. *Addiction*, **102**(11), 1711–1721.

Edwards, G., Gross, M.M., Keller, M., Moser, J., & Room, R. (Eds.). (1977). Alcohol-related disabilities. Geneva: WHO, p17.

Fletcher, C. M., & Horn, D. (1970). Smoking and health report to the twenty-third World Health Assembly. *WHO Chronicle*, **24**, 345–370.

Grant, M. (1993). The role of the World Health Organization in alcohol research. *Alcohol Health and Research World*, **17**(3), 187.

Jernigan, H., Monteiro, M., Room, R., & Saxena, S. (2000). Towards a global alcohol policy: alcohol, public health and the role of the WHO. *Bulletin of the World Health Organization*, **78**(4), 491–499.

Kramer, J. F., & Cameron, D. C. (1975). A manual on drug dependence. Geneva: WHO.

Lien, G., & Deland, K. (2011). Translating the WHO Framework Convention on Tobacco Control: can we use tobacco control as a model for other non-communicable diseases? *Public Health*, **125**(12), 847–853.

Mamudu, H.M., & Glant, S.A. (2009). Civil society and the negotiation of the Framework Convention on Tobacco Control. *Global Public Health*, **4**, 150–168.

McAllister, W. (2000). Drug diplomacy in the twentieth century: an international history. London: Routledge.

McCarthy, M. (2002). A brief history of the World Health Organization. *Lancet*, **360**(9340), 1111–1112.

Moser, J. (1980). Prevention of alcohol-related problems: an international review of preventive measures, policies and programmes. Toronto: Addiction Research Foundation.

Mackay, J. (2013). Conversation with Judith Mackay. Interview 107. *Addiction*, **108**, 1897–1904.

Moser, J. (1984). Conversation with Joy Moser. Interview 7. *British Journal of Addiction*, **79**, 355–363.

Rehm, J. (2013). Defining substance use disorders: do we really need more than heavy use? *Alcohol and Alcoholism*, **46**(8), 633–640.

Room, R. (1981). A farewell to alcoholism? a commentary on the WHO 1980 expert committee report. *British Journal of Addiction*, **76**, 115–123.

Room R. (1984). The World Health Organization and alcohol control. *British Journal of Addiction*, **79**, 85–92.

Room, R. (1997). Harm reduction, human rights and the WHO expert committee on drug dependence. In P. Erickson et al. (Eds.), Harm reduction: a new direction for drug policies and programs. Toronto: University of Toronto Press. 119–130.

Room, R. (1998). Alcohol and drug disorders in the International Classification of Diseases: a shifting kaleidoscope. *Drug and Alcohol Review*, **17**, 305–317.

Room, R. (2005). Alcohol and the World Health Organization: the ups and downs of two decades. *Nordisk Alkohol and Narkotikatidskrift*, **22**, 146–162.

Room, R. (2012). Conversation with Robin Room. Journal Interview 100. *Addiction*, **107**, 493–500.

Room, R., & Babor, T. (2005). World Health Organization's global action on alcohol: resources required to match the rhetoric. *Addiction*, **100**(5), 579–580.

Selvaggio, K. (1984). World Health Organization bottles up alcohol study. *International Journal of Health Services*, **14**(2), 303–388.

Taylor, A., & Bettcher, D. (2000). WHO Framework Convention on Tobacco Control: a global 'good' for public health. *Bulletin of the World Health Organization*, **78**, 920–929.

Weishaar, H., Collin, J., Smith, K., Grüning, T., Mandal, S., & Gilmore, A. (2012). Global health governance and the commercial sector: a documentary analysis of tobacco company strategies to influence the WHO Framework Convention on Tobacco Control. *PLoS Medicine*, **9**(6), e1001249.

World Health Organization. (1949). Expert Committee on Habit-Forming Drugs. Geneva: WHO.

World Health Organization. (1950). Expert Committee on Drugs Liable to Produce Addiction. Second report. WHO Technical Report Series 21. Geneva: WHO.

World Health Organization. (1951). Expert Committee on Mental Health, Alcoholism Subcommittee. First report. Technical Report Series 42. Geneva: WHO.

World Health Organization. (1952a). Expert Committee on Drugs Liable to Produce Addiction. Third report. Technical Report Series 5. Geneva: WHO.

World Health Organization. (1952b). Expert Committee on Mental Health, Alcoholism Subcommittee. Second report. Technical Report Series 48. Geneva: WHO.

World Health Organization. (1954). Expert Committee on Alcohol. First report. Geneva: WHO.

World Health Organization. (1955). Alcohol and alcoholism: report of an expert committee. Technical Report Series 94. Geneva: WHO.

World Health Organization. (1957). Expert Committee on Addiction-Producing Drugs. Seventh report. Technical Report Series 116. Geneva: WHO.

World Health Organization. (1958). Expert Committee on Addiction-Producing Drugs. Eighth report. Technical Report Series 142. Geneva: WHO.

World Health Organization. (1959). Expert Committee on Addiction-Producing Drugs. Ninth report. Technical Report Series 160. Geneva: WHO.

World Health Organization. (1960). Expert Committee on Addiction-Producing Drugs. Tenth report. Technical Report Series 188. Geneva: WHO.

World Health Organization. (1961). Expert Committee on Addiction-Producing Drugs. Eleventh report. Technical Report Series 211. Geneva: WHO.

World Health Organization. (1964). Expert Committee on Addiction-Producing Drugs. Twelfth report. Technical Report Series 273. Geneva: WHO.

World Health Organization. (1965). Expert Committee on Dependence-Producing Drugs. Fourteenth report. Technical Report Series 312. Geneva: WHO.

World Health Organization. (1967a). Expert Committee on Mental Health Services for the Prevention and Treatment of Dependence on Alcohol and Other Drugs. Technical Report Series 363. Geneva: WHO.

World Health Organization. (1967b). Expert Committee on Mental Health. Technical Report Series 367. Geneva: WHO.

World Health Organization. (1969). Expert Committee on Drug Dependence. Sixteenth report. Technical Report Series 407. Geneva: WHO.

World Health Organization. (1970). WHO Resolution WHA23.32. Health consequences of smoking.

World Health Organization. (1971). Director-General. The limitation of smoking. Report submitted to the twenty-fourth World Health Assembly. *WHO Chronicle*, **25**, 452–457.

World Health Organization. (1973). Expert Committee on Drug Dependence. Nineteenth report. Technical Report Series 526. Geneva: WHO.

World Health Organization. (1974). Expert Committee on Drug Dependence. Twentieth report. Technical Report Series 551. Geneva: WHO.

World Health Organization. (1975a). History of international public health. Geneva: WHO.

World Health Organization. (1975b). Smoking and its effects on health: report of a WHO Expert Committee. Geneva: WHO.

World Health Organization. (1979). Expert Committee on Smoking Control. Controlling the smoking epidemic: report of the WHO Expert Committee on Smoking Control. Geneva: WHO.

World Health Organization. (1993a). Expert Committee on Drug Dependence. WHO Technical Report Series 833. Geneva: WHO.

World Health Organization. (1993b). Expert Committee on Health Promotion in the Workplace. Alcohol and drug abuse. Technical Report Series 833. Geneva: WHO.

World Health Organization. (1994). Lexicon of alcohol and drug terms. Geneva: WHO.

World Health Organization. (1995a). Expert Committee on Drug Dependence. Twenty-ninth report. WHO Technical Report Series 856. Geneva: WHO.

World Health Organization. (1995b). WHO Resolution WHA.48.11. An international strategy for tobacco control.

World Health Organization. (1996). WHO Resolution WHA49.17. International Framework Convention for Tobacco Control.

World Health Organization. (1997). Strategy framework and work plan 1997. http://apps.who.int/iris/bitstream/10665/63317/1/WHO_MSA_PSA_97.2.pdf?ua=1

World Health Organization. (1998). Guidelines for controlling and monitoring the smoking epidemic. Geneva: WHO.

World Health Organization. (1999a). Expert Committee on Drug Dependence. Thirty-first report. Geneva: WHO.

World Health Organization. (1999b). Working Group on the WHO Framework Convention on Tobacco Control. Report of the first meeting of the working group. Geneva: WHO.

World Health Organization. (2003a). Expert Committee on Drug Dependence. Thirty-third report. Technical Report Series 915. Geneva: WHO.

World Health Organization. (2003b). Framework Convention on Tobacco Control. Geneva: WHO.

World Health Organization. (2005). WHO Resolution WHA58.26. Public health problems caused by harmful use of alcohol.

World Health Organization. (2007a). Expert Committee on Problems Related to Alcohol Consumption. Second report. Geneva: WHO.

World Health Organization. (2007b). Study Group on Tobacco Product Regulation. Report on the scientific basis of tobacco product regulation. Technical Report Series 945. Geneva: WHO.

World Health Organization. (2010). WHO Resolution WHA63.13. Global strategy to reduce the harmful use of alcohol.

Yach, D., & Bettcher, D. (1998). The globalization of public health. *American Journal of Public Health*, **88**, 735–774.

Yach, D., & Bettcher, D. (2000). Globalisation of tobacco industry influence and new global responses. *Tobacco Control*, **9**, 206–216.

Yach, D., & Monteiro, M.G. (2011). The road to a World Health Organization global strategy for reducing the harmful use of alcohol. *Alcohol Research & Health*, **34**(2), 257–260.

Chapter 5

The role of stakeholders in addictions policy and intervention

Esben Houborg, Betsy Thom, Franca Beccaria, Irmgard Eisenbach-Stangl, Rachel Herring, Jacek Moskalewicz, and Marta Welbel

5.1 Addiction policy

Addiction, and addiction policy, affect an increasing number of people, especially over recent decades when new types of behaviour have come to be conceptualized as addictions—excessive and repetitive shopping, gaming, surfing the Internet, using mobile phones, sex, physical training, to name a few. In this chapter we restrict ourselves to addiction to drugs and alcohol. The aim of the chapter is to present stakeholder theory and provide some examples of how it may be applied in the field of addiction policy. The paper arises from research conducted as part of the ALICE RAP project, a large transdisciplinary European programme (http://www.alicerap.eu). Case studies conducted in five countries (Austria, Italy, Denmark, Poland, and the United Kingdom) examined stakeholder dynamics and the relationships between stakeholders in the drug and alcohol policy arenas.

The chapter is divided into three main sections. The first section examines the stakeholder concept and presents different theoretical perspectives on stakeholders and stakeholding. The next section describes and discusses different types of stakeholders within the addiction policy field. The third part of the chapter illustrates key themes using case studies of stakeholding in substitution treatment from the five countries mentioned. It should be noted that the cases and examples do not necessarily involve policies and practices where the concept of 'addiction' figures or plays a significant role. They are more broadly about policies and practices that are directed at behavioural problems that involve drugs and alcohol and that are variously labelled as 'addiction', 'dependence', 'misuse', 'abuse', 'problematic use', and the like.

5.2 'Stakeholders': concepts and theories

The concept of 'stakeholder', and the initial development of stakeholder theory, is rooted in the business science literature (Clarkson, 1995; Freeman, 1984), but it has also become prominent within political and policy discourse since the 1990s. Stakeholder theory aimed to explain the relationship between an organization and its external environment. Freeman, writing from a business perspective, argued that apart from shareholders there are other parties related to a company whose interests need to be taken into account. He defined stakeholders as 'any group or individual who is affected by or who can affect the achievement of an organization's objectives' (Freeman, 1984, p. 46). Within this definition, a person, an informal group, an organization, or an institution may all be stakeholders. Brugha and Varasovsky (2000) adopt a similar broad definition for policy analysis. They define stakeholders 'as actors who have an interest in the issue under consideration, who are affected by the issue, or who—because of their position—have or should have an active or passive influence on the decision-making and implementation processes' (p. 341).

Stakeholder theory has generated much debate and has been criticized as vague and ambiguous (Fassin, 2009). There is no consensus as to what the concept of stakeholder means, with hundreds of definitions published (Miles, 2012; Wagner Mainardes et al., 2011). Who 'counts' as a stakeholder differs significantly depending upon the situation or the question at hand, but also on whether a narrow or broad definition is used. Those adopting a narrow definition have tended to emphasize the legitimacy of stakeholder claims, whereas those preferring broad definitions have stressed the stakeholder's power to influence an organization regardless of legitimacy (Mitchell et al., 1997).

5.3 Stakeholders' interests and representation

If the 'stake' that stakeholders have in a particular issue or policy—and which constitutes them as 'stakeholders'—is defined as 'interests', the stakeholder concept may be said to bear a close relationship to the concept of 'interest groups'. But the concept of interest group itself has different meanings. Beyers and colleagues (2008, p. 1103) define interest groups according to three factors: organization, political interests, and informality. Interest groups are thus organized forms of political behaviour that seek to influence policy, but without seeking political office (p. 1106). Beyers et al. distinguish between interest groups that are formed with the purpose of influencing policy, such as Greenpeace, and 'latent interest groups', such as sports clubs, that would normally not seek to influence policy, but may do so under particular circumstances (p. 1107). This definition of interest groups thus involves collective action in some manner in order to influence policy.

Interest groups have been classified in other ways under a variety of labels; for instance, groups may be classified according to their function into partial or sectional groups where the main goal is to protect the interests of members (e.g. trades organizations and professional associations) and into cause groups, interested in promoting a specific issue or cause (e.g. drug user rights, drug decriminalization). Walt (1994) discusses a further distinction between 'insider' groups—recognized and legitimized by government (e.g. Association of British Pharmaceutical Industry)—and 'outsider' groups, which do not enjoy the same level of legitimacy and may find it difficult to penetrate the policy process (e.g. drug user groups). This way of classifying groups rests on their relationship to decision-making authorities and their power to influence such authorities.

As indicated previously, interest groups are not necessarily defined according to their social position or particular attributes. They may also be defined according to a particular interest that people have in a policy or issue unrelated to their social position or personal attributes, such as concerns over environmental issues (Andersen et al., 1998, p. 113). This broader definition of interest groups has a close resemblance to the stakeholder concept as we have employed it: first, because 'interests' and 'stakes' may both be defined in relation to structural and other (individual) characteristics as well as to subjective opinions and attitudes; and second, because stakeholders and interest groups are not necessarily engaged in political behaviour. The latter point is important because there may be actors who are affected by a policy or an issue, but who cannot, will not, or do not contemplate engagement in political behaviour in order to influence policy. Alcoholics Anonymous and Narcotics Anonymous, for instance, are two such groups. Thus, what constitutes a stakeholder will always be an empirical question which demands investigation of how different actors affect and/or are affected by a policy. However, whatever the function or position of the group in relation to the policy process, it is important to have the structural dimension in mind when making a stakeholder analysis as it pertains to the issue of *power*.

5.4 **Power, interest, and influence**

A key distinction in the conceptualization of stakeholders is the distinction between stakeholders that *affect* a policy or an organization and stakeholders that are *affected*. The two are of course not mutually exclusive, but neither are they necessarily connected. Stakeholders may thus be affected by a policy without being able to affect it. This, of course, concerns issues of power and its distribution among stakeholders.

Mitchell et al. (1997) argued that all stakeholders possess some kind of combination of three critical attributes: *power, legitimacy*, and *urgency. Stakeholder salience*, 'the degree to which managers give priority to competing stakeholder claims' (p. 869), is viewed as positively related to the accumulative number of the three attributes of power, legitimacy, and urgency. Legitimacy and urgency tend to be dynamic rather than static; they are socially constructed and determined by perception rather than by objective reality. Stakeholders holding one or more of the three attributes may not be aware of them or may choose not to use them (Mitchell et al., 1997).

The power/interest matrix as presented by Ackermann and Eden (1998, 2011) (see Figure 5.1) is also relevant when translating stakeholder theory from business and management literature into the social sciences as it helps us distinguish between different stakeholders according to their power and their 'stake' in the issue at hand. Ackermann and Eden's matrix consists of four compartments based on the strength of stakeholders' power to influence the future of an

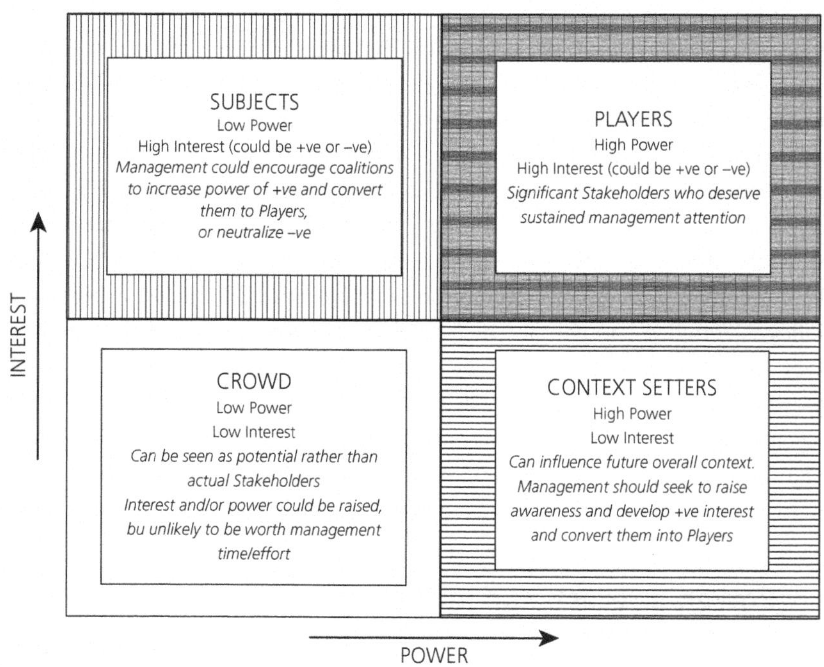

Fig. 5.1 Power/interest matrix.

Reprinted from *Long Range Planning*, 44, Ackermann, F. and Eden, C., Strategic Management of Stakeholders: Theory and Practice, 179–196. Copyright © 2011, with permission from Elsevier.

issue and on the degree of interest stakeholders have in the issue. In this way some stakeholders may be powerful and have a strong interest in the issue; these stakeholders are defined as *players*. Other stakeholders may be powerful, but have a weak interest in the issue; these stakeholders are defined as *context setters*. Yet other stakeholders may be less powerful, but have a strong interest in the issue; these are defined as *subjects*. Finally, some stakeholders may be less powerful and have a weak interest in the issue; they are defined as *crowd*.

In terms of the definition of stakeholders as actors that affect or are affected by a policy, this matrix helps us distinguish between stakeholders according to their power to affect the policy and the degree of their interest in relation to how they are affected. As Hellman (2012) discusses, current trends in the addictions field, especially in relation to alcohol, towards a multistakeholder approach to policy making highlight the importance of considering inequalities in the power position of different stakeholder groups. Multistakeholder approaches, she argues, require the incorporation of different rationalities, different understandings of the issues, and different beliefs about solutions into a consensus model of action which fails to take account of unequal political power.

Eden and Ackermann's as well as Mitchell's frameworks can be illustrated empirically by de Bussy and Kelly's (2010) study of the stakeholder concept in politics in Western Australia. The study identified a gap between politicians' comments about groups that they said that they *should* pay attention to in principle (i.e. legitimate stakeholders) and those that they *actually* paid attention to (i.e. salient stakeholders). The politicians gave more salience to stakeholders who held similar 'philosophical' beliefs to their own and to *organized groups* (e.g. industry groups, lobbyists, and NGOs) that were able to command the attention of policymakers. Other 'unorganized' groups with legitimate claims (e.g. young people, people with disabilities, and those living in remote areas) were marginalized by their lack of power. The authors concluded that 'in politics, legitimacy is the major determinant of stakeholder identification but power is the key to understanding stakeholder salience' (de Bussy & Kelly, 2010, p. 301).

In the addictions field, for instance, the history of professional involvement indicates the dynamic, socially constructed nature of policy salience at any particular point in time. Drug substitution treatment is one policy arena where different professional groups have vied for legitimacy and policy influence in championing or opposing policy responses (Beccaria et al., 2013). To take another example, substance users very often fall within a 'non-stakeholder' category and are seen as lying outside the policy arena. But, as Bjerge and her colleagues illustrate in Chapter 6 of this book, illicit drug users have taken action to gain a voice through acquiring the three attributes of power, legitimacy, and urgency described by Mitchell et al. (1997).

5.5 Stakeholders within the addictions policy field

Over the years, policy to regulate various aspects of drug and alcohol production and consumption has been shaped by many different interests and social actors—stakeholders (Sournia, 1990). For instance, historically, in many countries, especially those with a strong temperance movement, alcohol abuse or addiction was treated as a moral issue making social and penal institutions important stakeholders in alcohol policy. During the nineteenth century, medicine, in particular psychiatry, emerged as an institution of control to supervise troublesome individuals, in institutions such as asylums, where the mentally ill, the poor, or 'inebriates'—the term used at the time for people with an alcohol problem—were detained in 'treatment' for indeterminate periods of time (Levine, 1978; McLaughlin, 1991).

More recently, particularly since the 1960s and 1970s, when the modern drug problem developed, addiction has become an issue that involves many different kinds of stakeholders from different sectors of society. For example, because drug and alcohol addiction came to be understood as a learned behaviour, psychologists and social workers employed in both public and private organizations came to play an important role in the treatment field in many countries, including Denmark, Sweden, and the UK.

In contemporary times, public health practitioners, epidemiologists, and public health researchers have entered the picture and turned the focus of attention to the behaviour of the population as a whole. In many countries, because dependence or addiction emerged as a medical problem, it was mainly managed within the medical community by doctors and medico-administrative institutions such as national boards of health (Berridge, 1979, 1984; Edman, 2012, 2013; Houborg, 2014a), although penal institutions continued to play a prominent part in national responses. In some countries, like the United States and Finland, however, there is also a long tradition of managing the problems to a great degree outside the medical system; for example, by adopting policies which restrict availability (through alcohol monopolies and taxes) or through civic society movements, including the particularly influential movement Alcoholic Anonymous (AA) and its equivalent for drug users, Narcotics Anonymous (NA). In the United States, for instance, addiction problems are typically dealt with in small civic communities and support group systems, an approach which has been strong in countries with a weak or residual welfare state. As Hellman and Room (2014) have argued, 'The features of the AA solution, with the key factors of voluntariness, personal initiative and resourcefulness, are a good fit with the US residual welfare state' (pp. 2–3). In Finland, on the other hand, 'The inclusive strategies of substance use policies, prevention, and treatment follow the basic rationale of the Nordic social democratic welfare state'. The comparison highlights the relevance of how 'addiction' is framed and translated into policy action within different state welfare systems to the engagement of different groups of actors as the principal players in policy formation and implementation.

Policies dealing with the treatment, prevention, and control of addiction are constantly developing and changing, for several reasons. One is the desire to grasp, explain, and conceptualize the changing and varying behavioural problems related to alcohol and drugs. The fact that some people seem to lose control over their own actions in relation to these substances has proved to be a tricky epistemological issue, resulting in the constant emergence and evolution of different medical, psychological, and sociological explanations. This is also why researchers and others involved in the processes of framing and reframing how we think about the use and misuse of drugs and alcohol play such an important part as stakeholders in addictions policy.

Another reason for the shifts in addictions policy is that new problems and new kinds of people with problems constantly appear. For example, during the 1960s, substances such as cannabis and LSD were introduced in some countries and new groups of people started to use them; during the 1980s and 1990s, ecstasy became an important issue in many countries. Sometimes new problems arise from the unintended consequences of existing policies, such as risks and consequences associated with the criminalization of drug use. A good example of this is the issue of new psychoactive substances, the so-called legal highs, which are alternatives to illicit drugs and which contain ingredients developed to evade restrictions related to the growing list of prohibited substances named in international drug control conventions. The European Monitoring Centre for Drugs and Drug Addiction (EMCDDA) reported in 2015 that there had been a sevenfold increase in seizures of new psychoactive substances between 2008 and 2013, and that in 2014 a record 101 new psychoactive substances were recorded for the first time (EMCDDA, 2015, p. 4).

Thus the marketing of new drugs or the framing of behaviours, such as 'binge drinking', as a policy-relevant problem influences policy responses. New groups emerge advocating claims for what they want to be taken into account in addictions policy, sometimes with success sometimes without. For example, during the 1970s and 1980s, some parents of drug users in Denmark vigorously campaigned to get drug problems recognized as a medical condition that could be treated with methadone. They were unsuccessful, and in the end it was not until the National Council on Drugs shifted its position in the mid-1980s that methadone maintenance treatment was accepted in Denmark (Houborg, 2013).

This shows that even though people are affected by drug problems and drug policies, and express a common view as a group—and hence can be considered stakeholders or interest groups with regard to drug policy—their interests and concerns may not, in the end, be taken into account in the policy-making process.

Furthermore, in some cases, problems, concerns, and interests may remain unarticulated. While it may be stretching the concept of stakeholder too far to see such groups (the 'crowd') as having an interest, nevertheless circumstances may change the position and engagement of these 'invisible' or 'crowd' stakeholders and prompt more active involvement in the policy process at one time or another. Sometimes a window of opportunity may open that makes it possible for particular concerns and problems to be taken into account and for new stakeholders to enter the arena of policymaking.

An example is the entry of drug users—formerly an 'invisible' stakeholder group—into the policy arena. In Denmark during the 1990s, drug users were able to enter the drug policy arena as an organized interest group (Houborg, 2012; Bjerge et al., Chapter 6 in this volume). Briefly, social policy reforms during the 1990s had led to a focus on social exclusion and, as drug users were perceived as a marginalized group, one initiative was to support the organization of drug users. The Narcotics Council that advises the government on drug issues started to include the organized drug users as a stakeholder in their activities and writing. In this way, a place was carved out for drug users to articulate their own interests and concerns about drug policy. In another example, from the UK, a number of factors came together to allow critics of methadone maintenance treatment to advocate a 'recovery' approach with a goal of drug abstinence. The ensuing debate did not result in a radical policy shift, but it did prompt reconsideration of treatment aims and resulted in changes in the treatment system (Duke et al., 2013).

The emergence of new stakeholders and opportunities are especially visible in countries which experienced systemic transitions. The shift in alcohol policy in Poland in the 1990s is a good example. In the early 1980s, Poland implemented a comprehensive system of alcohol policy based on the Nordic model, with a variety of control measures on alcohol consumption and treatment interventions as complementary measures. Its provisions were included in the Law on Upbringing in Sobriety and Counteracting Alcoholism of 1982 and were a result of a consensus between the authorities and a new stakeholder—the first in the socialist block—the independent trade union movement Solidarity. After a few years, Poland became a scene of rapid political and economic changes, including transition from a centrally controlled economy to a free market system. As the state alcohol monopoly was broken, new stakeholders emerged, including those engaged in the production, distribution, and sale of alcohol. This group consisted of a variety of participants—from private importers and small shop owners to huge international companies. They had a strong economic interest in changing the existing alcohol policy and soon became a powerful stakeholder in this field. The social and political climate was favourable to changes too, as all solutions based on control measures were associated with the 'old regime'. Within the next years, a shift in alcohol policy was clearly noticeable—most of the control measures were abolished step-by-step and emphasis was put on treatment and preventive education programmes addressed to school children and youngsters (Moskalewicz, 1993; Moskalewicz & Simpura, 2000; Świątkiewicz & Wieczorek, 2009).

Thus, as patterns of drug use change and policy designed to address the problems of drug or alcohol use influences new behaviour patterns, the composition and influence of stakeholders vary and change. The previous examples illustrate the need to map out stakeholders and contextualize their activities within the different national cultures and the political, health, and social systems in force at particular points in time.

5.6 **Institutions, professionals, and experts as stakeholders**

Drug and alcohol policy is often conceptualized as constituted of four different policy areas: regulation/control, prevention, treatment, and harm reduction. This means that a number of different public and private institutions and organizations are involved in alcohol and drug policy and hence have the potential to influence addiction policy. Furthermore, the way in which drug and alcohol policy frames the balance between regulation and control, on the one hand, and treatment, prevention, and harm reduction, on the other, is also important for addiction policy.

Stakeholders at different levels of policy formation and implementation may have very different ideas about how the perceived problem should—or, in practical terms, can—be addressed. For example, in Denmark a zero-tolerance policy on possession of illicit drugs was introduced in 2004. However, this policy included an exemption for people with addiction problems who have limited financial resources: they could receive a caution instead of a fine when caught in possession of illicit drugs. More or less similar policies can be found in other countries where policies and measures are designed to divert people with addiction problems from punishment to treatment (e.g. through drug courts in the U.S.). In this case criminal justice policy in relation to illicit drugs and policy concerned with the health aspects of addiction get entangled, and stakeholders in the criminal justice system play an important part as stakeholders in addiction policy. This can be further emphasized when looking at the implementation of zero-tolerance policy in Denmark. Even though Danish legislation makes it possible to exempt poor drug addicts from punishment, research has shown that in fact the implementation of zero-tolerance policy this provision is rarely used (Houborg, 2014b). Rather, the police seem to emphasize zero tolerance over consideration for drug addicts when implementing the legislation.

There are specific areas of addiction policy that clearly need the cooperation of stakeholders from different domains; for example, the provision of drug addiction treatment in detention and prison. Alcohol issues also cross government departments and policy domains. Often the same stakeholders are engaged in policy regarding the health aspects of consumption and the criminal justice aspects of problem drinking or 'binge drinking'. For instance, drunk drivers in the UK may be offered the chance to attend driver education classes as an alternative to prison. Sometimes such cooperation can bring unexpected results, as stakeholders from different government departments can present different approaches to specific solutions. For example, in Poland, where development of methadone maintenance treatment (MMT) progressed rather slowly, in penitentiary units it developed quite quickly after 2005. Recommendations in 2009 clarified that every opioid-dependent person in prison should have access to MMT as well as a choice between such treatment and drug-free therapy. As a consequence, in 2011 about 15 per cent of MMT patients consisted of those receiving this treatment within the in-prison programmes (Moskalewicz & Welbel, 2013).

As noted already, the history of addictions policy varies from country to country. There are differences with regard to which public institutions and organizations and which parts of the political system and the administrative apparatus influence addictions policy. Over time, there are also changes in which parts of the public sector play the main stakeholder role. In Denmark, for example, the healthcare system was the main stakeholder in drug addiction policy until the 1960s when a change of policy occurred; the emergence of the new drug problem associated with the new youth culture resulted in the social welfare system becoming the main stakeholder. On the other hand, with regard to alcohol addiction, it was mainly the social welfare and criminal justice systems that were the main stakeholders for many years until the problem was reframed as a medical issue, with the result that today, the healthcare system is the main stakeholder.

In contrast, in Italy the healthcare system became the main stakeholder in drug addiction only during the 1990s, because of the challenge posed by the AIDS epidemic. Before then, drug addiction was considered mainly a moral and educational problem and was treated in therapeutic communities without the use of prescribed drugs (Beccaria & Rolando, 2013). Wine production has always played an important role in the Italian economy, making alcohol producers important stakeholders; wine culture has downplayed alcohol-related problems. Until 2001, alcohol addiction was never the subject of specific laws and, with the exception of self-help groups, specific treatment services did not exist before the 1990s (Beccaria & Roland, 2014).

Usually the conceptualization of addiction dominant in an individual country determines which sector is engaged in developing and implementing addiction policy. Two examples from Poland illustrate the importance of problem conceptualization for stakeholder saliency.

In the nineteenth and early twentieth centuries in Poland, as in many other countries, the moral model was dominant in relation to alcohol misuse. As a result, users were seen as weak, antisocial, and deserving of condemnation; the criminal justice system was the main stakeholder in the field. Since the mid-1950s, when the medical model became dominant, the healthcare sector began to play the most important role, introducing drug antagonist medication as the most relevant intervention. In the 1990s, the public health context was neglected as a model underlining individual problems and needs became dominant. At the same time, an important stakeholder in alcohol policy emerged—the State Agency for Solving Alcohol Problems—and from that time it has become a key stakeholder with the task of bringing together different domains and sectors important for alcohol policy.

Changes in stakeholders and public sector domains engaged in drug policy in Poland were also a result of shifts in approaches to illicit drugs. *The Act on Prevention of Drug Abuse* of 1985 developed a system based on drug demand reduction; the possession of any amount of drugs was not penalized. In the late 1990s, that approach changed: policy towards drug users became the domain of the criminal justice system. Legislative acts of 1997 and 2000, step-by-step, criminalized the problem of substance use; possession of even the smallest amount of any narcotic drug was penalized and the possibility of referring users to treatment services instead of prison was limited. Criticism of these restrictive solutions came from stakeholders and experts from different fields, and in 2011 an amendment was made which introduced the possibility of discontinuance of proceedings towards drug users who possessed drugs only for their own use. However, this amendment neither depenalized drug possession nor changed the criminal justice–oriented approach that has dominated in Poland since 1997 (Moskalewicz & Welbel, 2013; Olszewska, 2011).

Thus as the field of addictions grew in the late twentieth century, experts and researchers from an increasing range of disciplines entered the field—from medicine, social work, psychology, pharmacology, criminology, public health, and epidemiology. User groups also entered the arena and some stakeholders banded together in coalitions to improve their chances of influencing policy in the desired direction. The professional and institutional links of those involved in addictions policy, prevention, and treatment activity meant that a far greater number of institutions and agencies were drawn into the stakeholder arena, introducing an increasing complex—and at times conflictual—dynamic into policymaking.

5.7 Civic society and corporate stakeholders

Individuals experiencing addiction or drug- and alcohol-related problems are clearly an important target for policy measures and, as such, can be seen as stakeholders, albeit, in Ackermann and Eden's (2011) terms, they are very often the 'crowd' or 'subjects' with low engagement in policy. Equally, also part of the 'crowd', there are the stakeholders such as family, relatives, and friends who experience problems in relation to addiction problems and hence are affected by the policies and measures directed at users. In addition, the repercussions of drug and alcohol use can spread to local communities that are affected by drug scenes, businesses that are concerned about alcohol problems among employees, and town centres disrupted by heavy drinking in the night-time economy. Although often invisible and silent, such private stakeholders can affect policy. It is significant that in relation to both drug and alcohol use, private actors have succeeded in raising claims, representing organized interests, and developing responses towards addiction. The AA movement and equivalent organizations with regard to drugs, although not generally visible participants in the policy process, play an important role. In some countries, such as Iceland, the AA movement has had a significant impact on addiction policy. In Italy, Clubs of Alcohol Treatment (CAT) played the major role in creating a public arena around alcohol problems at the end of the twentieth century; they succeeded in establishing an alliance with professionals working in local addiction services (Beccaria & Rolando, 2014). Privately run therapeutic communities and private practitioners have played a role in developing drug and alcohol treatment in countries such as Denmark and the UK. Denmark, Sweden, Finland, and Poland also provide good examples of countries where nonstate (NGOs) as well as public-private collaborations have played important roles in responding to drug and alcohol problems. In fact, in Poland, NGOs—which arose from a therapeutic community approach—managed to dominate the healthcare system in relation to drug addiction therapy (Świątkiewicz et al., 1998).

The field of addiction policy, and policy towards drugs and alcohol more generally, is thus a field where policy is not solely, or even mainly, associated with *government* policy, but rather has developed through various forms of interaction, collaboration, and negotiation between public and private actors. This means that addiction policy is an area where *governance*, understood as policy-making and implementation through public-private collaboration and networks, has played and continues to play an important role.

Currently, corporate stakeholders constitute perhaps the most influential group of private stakeholders in alcohol policies. Their position has grown particularly since the 1990s, illustrated by the fact that countries of the Soviet bloc underwent a transition towards market economies and Nordic alcohol monopolies were reduced to retail level. Prior to those times in these countries, both private and state-owned alcohol industries, although important stakeholders, had their interests restricted by public health and order considerations. The establishment of the World Trade Organization, other international trade agreements, and economic integration occurring in different regions of the world stimulated the further growth of multinational industries and opened avenues of expansion into new market economies and emerging markets in developing countries (Moskalewicz &Wieczorek, in press, 2016). As the new post-1990 economic order treated alcohol as any other commodity, restrictive alcohol policies had to be relaxed and domestic markets with restrictive access had to be opened to the international alcohol industry (Grieshaber-Otto et al., 2000; Zeigler, 2009). A window for expansion was opened up for corporate stakeholders by powerful global economic stakeholders whose aim was general liberalization and the removal of barriers for economic activities (Jernigan, 2012). New economic opportunities were very much welcomed and immediately exploited by stakeholders from the alcohol industry. They affected the development of liberal alcohol policies not only in countries in transition towards a market economy (Moskalewicz & Simpura, 2000) and in emerging economies in developing countries (Odejide, 2006), but also broke traditional Nordic alcohol policies (Ugland, 2002). Corporate stakeholders also influenced better-off countries such as Switzerland and Japan to reduce customs duties on imported beverages (Zeigler, 2009). As a result of economic globalization, alcohol production increased enormously and quickly underwent consolidation. By the end of the first decade of the twenty-first century, the global alcohol market was worth almost US $1trillion, of which around $500 billion belonged to beer companies (Jernigan, 2012). Almost half of globalized sales of alcohol by volume were attributable to only ten global producers (International Center for Alcohol Policies, 2006). Thus, even within the group of corporate stakeholders, some emerged as more powerful than others.

Corporate stakeholders have become increasingly recognized as partners in international debates on alcohol policy and in multistakeholder approaches to policy (Hellman, 2012). They have been able to influence international public health stakeholders such as the World Health Organization (WHO), which reframed its goal from reducing overall alcohol consumption to reducing harmful alcohol consumption. Moreover, WHO, in its resolution from the fifty-eighth World Health Assembly, encourages member states to open consultations with representatives of the industry in order to limit the health impact of harmful alcohol consumption (WHO, 2005,).

Experiences of the last three decades, summarized in this section, show how corporate alcohol stakeholders—which Eden and Ackermann (1998) would describe as *subjects*—initially with strong interest, but relatively less power, have exploited opportunities created by global economic transformations. They could also be described as *context setters* who, in a relatively short time, achieved a position as major *players* with strong interests related to growing alcohol consumption worldwide and with great power to satisfy these interests.

5.8 **Stakeholders in opioid substitution treatment policy**

In this section we illustrate some of the themes discussed earlier, using examples from case studies of opioid substitution treatment policy conducted in Poland, Italy, Denmark, the UK, and Finland. Kingdon's (1984) theory provides the theoretical framework for these case studies. They illustrate, and allow comparison of, ways in which stakeholder positioning, legitimacy, and power can be affected by political change, and also how stakeholder groups can use shifts in political systems and policy approaches to further their interests.

As noted earlier, changes in the political, social, or economic context can create an opportunity for stakeholder activity to influence policy. One case study showed how the introduction and development of MMT came about in Poland during the 1990s, mainly as a result of concerns about HIV and the economic and political changes that occurred in Poland during this period (Moskalewicz & Welbel, 2013). The study identified a large number of stakeholders that were engaged in the issue, mainly public and private institutions at local, national, and international levels, as well as cross-situational organized interests. The following stakeholders were included in the study: policy-makers and politicians at regional and local levels; treatment providers and professional groups; NGOs representing users, their families, harm-reduction activists, therapeutic services, church associations, and the like; scientists and researchers; media and public opinion representatives; as well as international bodies such as the WHO, EMCDDA, and the United Nations Office on Drugs and Crime.

The study concluded that the window of opportunity for MMT, opening in the 1990s, soon closed, as stakeholders opposed to MMT gained salience and as the political climate conducive to such solutions changed when more restrictive legislation towards illicit drug-related problems was adopted in 1997. The main opposing stakeholders were organizations representing the well-established therapeutic community treatment approach, as well as regional politicians and local officials who were concerned about the conservative views of their voters and the rhetoric of the Catholic church proponents of MMT included professional groups, NGOs, and international organizations. International stakeholders played an important role as they provided training and expertise for MMT specialists, researchers, and other professionals, and issued recommendations which Poland, as a country aspiring to join different international structures, including the EU, had to take into consideration.

In Italy, where the influence of the Catholic church is just as high as in Poland, MMT has been hindered as well. The position of the church against the use of prescribed drugs in addiction treatment was exploited by advocates of therapeutic communities—most of them run by religious leaders—and by right-wing politicians. However, as in Poland and elsewhere, the HIV epidemic during the 1990s opened the policy window in which other stakeholders—mainly medical doctors and epidemiologists—were able to build consensus around the harm-reduction approach (Beccaria & Rolando, 2013).

In Denmark, MMT has a history dating back to the mid-1980s as part of a drug treatment policy with a strong emphasis on psychosocial treatment. The Danish case study, taking its point of departure in Kingdon's (1984) theory of policy change, showed that during the first decade of the twenty-first century there was a growing medicalization of Danish drug treatment policy. The study showed how addiction doctors, the National Board of Health, politicians, and administrators with a concern about the poor health state of Danish drug users played an important role in putting medical and health issues on the agenda. The study also showed how drug users increasingly came to be recognized as stakeholders in drug policy (Asmussen Frank et al., 2013).

A case study of the 'recovery' debate in the UK from the mid-2000s examined the ways in which opioid substitution treatment (OST), particularly methadone maintenance, was challenged and defended by key stakeholders in the initial phases of policy development and how they negotiated a 'recovery' focus as the organizing concept for British drug treatment policy from 2010. The study showed how some key stakeholders seized the opportunity presented by a 'policy window' to argue for a new strategy based on an abstinence-based, recovery-oriented framework. However, it also highlighted how stakeholders such as civil servants and government advisers, although less visibly engaged in the debates around MMT, played key roles in moderating the debates around the role of OST and in ensuring that an extreme policy of total abstinence did not appear in the published drug strategy document (Duke et al., 2013).

These case studies provide insight into the strategies stakeholder groups employ in attempting to position themselves in the policy arena and increase their policy salience. Contrary to the Polish and Italian cases, a Finnish case study showed the rapid development of opioid maintenance treatment in Finland from the 1990s. This study used Boltanski and Thévenot's (2006) theory of justification to analyze stakeholder salience and particularly the legitimacy of stakeholder claims. The issue of policy saliency was well illustrated. Not only professional (medical), but also cost efficiency claims concerning drug treatment were found to be of prime importance. The latter, mainly articulated by municipalities and other stakeholders who funded OST, gained salience (Perälä et al., 2013).

The case studies of OST policy focus on national policy and organized cross-situational interests and stakeholders (in some cases with international influences). Other case studies have been conducted that focus on local issues and situational stakeholders. One such study examines policies concerning the drug scene in a neighbourhood in Copenhagen (Houborg & Frank, 2014). In this case, different parts of civil society became engaged as more or less temporary stakeholders around specific issues and concerns, along with more established stakeholders such as NGOs, police, and municipal authorities. For example, some residents became temporarily engaged as drug policy stakeholders in order to influence measures directed towards the drug scene. Some residents were concerned with crime, disorder, and personal security, and wanted increased police efforts. Other residents wanted to develop measures and services for drug users that would minimize harms related to drugs and reduce the problems that the drug scene caused for the local community. Without institutionalized channels of influence or an established organized interest, the first group of residents found it difficult to have their concerns and interests recognized as legitimate claims in the policy process. The second group of residents, however, worked with drug policy activists, NGOs, and businesses, and organized to articulate their interests and concerns. This group was more successful in influencing the policy process. This case shows that stakeholders that are affected by a policy or an issue are not necessarily recognized as having legitimate claims on policy, and that it is particularly difficult to achieve salience if interests and concerns have not previously been organized.

Similarly, in Italy during the 1990s, drug users played an informal role at the local level in developing treatment services, but have always been absent as policy stakeholders (Beccaria & Rolando 2013; see also Bjerge et al., Chapter 6 in this book). The lack of drug user associations is seen to be related to the stigmatization of drug use—deeply rooted in the Italian culture under the influence of the Catholic church—showing that many variables can explain stakeholder salience or the absence of it, even, in some instances, stakeholders' 'self-exclusion'. However, changes occurring in drug consumption can always have an impact on the different stakeholders' positions within the policy arena. For example, the current prevalence of cannabis users among Italian drug users, along with the process of normalization of cannabis use, could result in increased salience of drug users in Italian drug politics (Chapter 6).

5.9 The relevance of the stakeholder concept

As mentioned earlier, the number of addictions is growing as more and more behavioural problems are problematized and conceived of in terms of addiction. This also means that increasing numbers of people engage in collective action around the problem of addiction, and this, in turn, entails an increase in the number of private and public organizations and institutions becoming stakeholders in addictions policy. Furthermore, involvement in addictions policy is also growing at municipal and local levels so that many more local organizations and agencies are drawn into the stakeholder arena. For instance, private organizations and businesses become concerned about addiction and develop policies and measures to address substance-related problems within their own agencies and in the local community. In some countries, we see how many private companies and other organizations, such as sports clubs or workplaces, have developed policies in relation to alcohol and drugs in recent years. Against this background, stakeholder analysis is a relevant and useful tool, increasing our understanding of how issues get onto the policy agenda and of the factors that influence policy formulation and implementation processes.

As should be clear from this chapter, addiction and addiction policy affect and are affected by many different actors, both directly and indirectly. The adoption of a broad definition of stakeholders as actors that affect or are affected by a policy issue draws attention to the fact that the voices heard in policy debates are not necessarily representative of all relevant groups at any particular time. As discussed here, not all relevant stakeholders are necessarily included as part of the public that is taken into account and given salience in policy debates and in the policy process. Stakeholder analysis highlights how policy is formulated and implemented. It reveals the strategies by which different groups of actors strive to position themselves favourably within the policy arena so that they may gain legitimacy for their preferred policy options and interests; it illustrates the contexts within which stakeholders emerge, survive, or disappear from the policy arena, and it identifies the factors which grant policy salience to some stakeholder groups, while others may be marginalized or excluded completely from the policy-making process.

References

Ackermann, F., & Eden, C. (2011). Strategic management of stakeholders: theory and practice. *Long Range Planning*, **44**, 179–196.

Andersen, H., Brante, T., & Korsnes, O. (1998). Leksikon i sociologi [Encyclopedia of sociology]. Copenhagen: Akademisk Forlag.

Asmussen Frank V., Bjerge B., & Houborg E. (2013). Shifts in opioid substitution treatment policy in Denmark from 2000–2011. *Substance Use & Misuse*, **48**, 997–1009.

Beccaria, F., Einstein, S., & Thom, B. (Eds.) (2013). Stakeholders in substitution treatment in six European countries *Substance Use & Misuse* [special issue], **48**(11).

Beccaria, F., & Rolando, S. (2013). Stakeholders' role in contemporary 'substitute drug' prescribing policies in Italy. *Substance Use & Misuse*, **48**, 943–953

Beccaria, F., & Rolando, S. (2014). The Italian politics of alcohol: the creation of a public arena at the end of the 20th century. *International Journal of Drug Policy* **26**(7), 662–669.

Berridge, V. (1979). Morality and medical science: concepts of narcotic addiction in Britain, 1820–1926. *Annals of Science*, **36**, 67–85.

Berridge, V. (1984). Drugs and social policy: the establishment of drug control in Britain 1900–1930. *British Journal of Addiction*, **79**, 17–29.

Beyers, J., Eising, R. and Maloney, W. (2008) Researching interest group politics in Europe and elsewhere: Much we study, little we know? *West European Politics* **31** (6): 1103–1128

Boltanski, L., & Thévenot, L. (2006). On justification: economies of worth. Princeton, NJ: Princeton University Press.

Brugha, R., & Varasovsky, Z. (2000). Stakeholder analysis; a review. *Health Policy and Planning*, **15**(3), 239–246.

Clarkson, M.B.E. (1995) A stakeholder framework for analyzing and evaluating corporate social performance. *Academy of Management Review* **20**(1), 92–117.

de Bussy, N., & Kelly, L. (2010). Stakeholders, politics and power: towards an understanding of stakeholder identification and salience in government. *Journal of Communications Management*, **14**(4), 289–305.

Duke, K., Herring, R., Thickett, A., & Thom, B. (2013). Substitute treatment in the era of 'recovery': an analysis of stakeholder roles and policy windows in Britain. *Substance Use & Misuse*, **48**(11), 996–976.

Duke, K., & Thom, B. (2014). The role of evidence and the expert in contemporary processes of governance: the case of opioid substitution treatment policy in England *International Journal of Drug Policy*. http://dx.doi.org/10.1016/j.drugpo.2014.01.015

Eden, C., & Ackermann, F. (1998). Making strategy: the journey of strategic management. London: Sage.

Edman, J. (2012). "Swedish drug treatment and the political use of conceptual innovation 1882–1982." Contemp. Drug Probs. **39**: 429.

Edman, J. (2013). The Ideological Drug Problem. *Drugs and Alcohol Today*, vol **13**, no. 1: 9–19.

EMCDDA. (2015, March). New psychoactive substances in Europe: an update from the EU Early Warning System. Lisbon: EMCDDA.

Fassin, Y. (2009). The stakeholder model refined. *Journal of Business Ethics*, **84**, 113–135.

Freeman, R.E. (1984). Strategic management: a stakeholder approach. Boston, MA: Pitman.

Grieshaber-Otto, J., Sinclair, S., & Schacter, N. (2000). Impacts of international trade, services and investment treaties on alcohol regulation. *Addiction*, **95**(12s4), 491–504.

Hellman, M. (2012). Multistakeholder alcohol policy: goal-based and value-based rationalities in an alcohol marketing task force In M. Hellman et al. (Eds.), A welfare policy patchwork: negotiating the public good in times of transition. Helsinki: Nordic Center for Welfare and Social Issues. 143–161.

Hellman, M., & Room, R. (2014). What's the story on addiction? Popular myths in the USA and Finland. *Critical Public Health*. http://dx.doi.org/10.1080/09581596.2014.926308

Houborg, E. (2012). The political pharmacology of methadone and heroin in Danish drug policy. *Contemporary Drug Problems*, **39**(Spring), 155–192.

Houborg, E. (2013). Methadone, a contested substance: Danish methadone policy in the 1970s. *International Journal of Drug Policy*, **24**, e73–e80.

Houborg, E. (2014a). Construction and handling of drug problems in Denmark from the 1870s to the 1980s. *Nordic Studies on Alcohol and Drugs*, **31**(5–6), 527–550.

Houborg, E. (2014b). Stofbrug og straf i Danmark [Drug use and punishment in Denmark]. *Gränsløs*, **1**(3), 27–35.

Houborg, E., & Frank, V. A. (2014). Drug consumption rooms and the role of governance and politics in policy processes. *International Journal of Drug Policy*, **25**(5), 972–977.

Houborg, E., Frank, V. A., & Bjerge, B. (2014). From zero-tolerance to non-enforcement: creating a new space for drug policing in Copenhagen, Denmark. *Contemporary Drug Problems*, **41**(Summer), 261–291.

International Center for Alcohol Policies (ICAP). (2006). The structure of the beverage alcohol industry. Report 17. Washington, DC: ICAP.

Jernigan, D. (2012). Global alcohol producers, science and policy: the case of the international centre for alcohol policies. *American Journal of Public Health*, **102**(1), 80–89.

Kim, J-N., Lan, N., & Sha, B-L. (2008). Breaking down the stakeholder environment: explicating approaches to the segmentation of publics for public relations research. *Journalism & Mass Communication Quarterly*, **85**(4), 751–768.

Kingdon, J. W. (1984). Policies agendas, alternatives, and public policies. Boston: Little, Brown.

Klingemann, J. (2013). Illusion of evidence based social policy. *Normy, dewiacje i kontrola społeczna*, **16**, 139–155.

Levine, H. (1978). The discovery of addiction: changing conceptions of habitual drunkenness in America. *Journal of Studies on Alcohol*, **39**(1), 143–74

Marres, N. (2007). The issues deserve more credit: pragmatist contributions to the study of public involvement in controversy. *Social Studies of Science*, **37**(5), 759–780.

McLaughlin, P. (1991). Inebriate reformatories in Scotland: an institutional history. In S. Barrows & R. Room (Eds.), Drinking: behavior and belief in modern history. Berkeley: University of California Press.

Miles, S. (2012). Stakeholder: essentially contested or just confused? *Journal of Business Ethics*, **108**, 285–298.

Mitchell, R.K., Agle, B.R., & Wood, D.J. (1997). Toward a theory of stakeholder identification and salience: defining the principle of who and what really counts. *Academy of Management Review*, **22**, 853–886

Moskalewicz, J. (1993). Lessons to be learnt from Poland's attempts at moderating its consumption of alcohol. *Addiction*, **88**(Suppl), 135–142.

Moskalewicz, J., & Simpura, J. (2000). The supply of alcoholic beverages in transitional conditions: the case of Central and Eastern Europe. *Addiction*, **95**(Suppl 4), S505–S522.

Moskalewicz, J., & Welbel, M. (2013). Walking through mud: history of the Polish methadone maintenance treatment from its stakeholders' perspective. *Substance Use & Misuse*, **48**(11), 977–996. doi: 10.3109/10826084.2013.797836.

Moskalewicz, J., & Wieczorek, Ł. (in press, 2016). Legal economies: the role of the alcohol industry. In T. Kolind et al., (Eds.), Handbook of drug and alcohol studies. London: Sage.

Odejide, O. (2006). Alcohol policies in Africa. *African Journal of Drug & Alcohol Studies*, **5**(1), 27–39.

Olszewska, W. (2011). Punishment for dealers, treatment for addicts. *Na wokandzie*, **6**. Accessed 12 March 2015. http://nawokandzie.ms.gov.pl/numer-6/wokanda-6/dilerow-karac-uzaleznionych-leczyc.html

Perälä R., Hellman, M., & Leppo, A. (2013). Behind the scenes: the justifications for opioid maintenance treatment in Finland. *Substance Use & Misuse*, **48**, 954–965.

Sournia, J.-C. (1990). A history of alcoholism. London: Blackwell.

Świątkiewicz, G., Moskalewicz, J., & Sierosławski, J. (1998). Therapeutic communities as a major response to drug problem in Poland. In H. Klingemann & G. Hunt (Eds.), Drugs, demons, and delinquents: drug treatment systems in international perspective. Thousand Oaks, CA: Sage. pp. 124–142

Świątkiewicz, G., & Wieczorek, Ł. (2009). Evolution of legal regulations concerning the alcohol supply in Poland from 1982 to 2005. *Alkoholizm i Narkomania*, **22**(3), 223–242.

Ugland, T. (2002). Policy re-categorization and integration: Europeanization of Nordic alcohol control policies. Oslo: ARENA Report No. 3 and SIRUS Report No. 1.

WHO. (2005). WHA58.26. Public-health problems caused by harmful use of alcohol: the fifty-eighth World Health Assembly. http://www.who.int/substance_abuse/wha_resolution_58_26_public_health_problems_alcohol.pdf

Wagner Mainardes, E., Alves, H., & Raposo, M. (2011). Stakeholder theory: issues to resolve. *Management Decision*, **49**(2), 226–252.

Walt, G. (1994). Health policy: an introduction to process and power. London: Zed Books.

Zeigler, D. (2009). The alcohol industry and trade agreements: a preliminary assessment. *Addiction*, **104**, 13–26.

Chapter 6

Exploring user groups as stakeholders in drug policy processes in four European countries

Bagga Bjerge, Karen Duke, Vibeke Asmussen Frank, Sara Rolando, and Irmgard Eisenbach-Stangl

6.1 User groups as stakeholders

This chapter discusses drug user groups as stakeholders in drug policy developments; more precisely, how drug user[1] groups act and get the opportunity to participate in policy processes. Inspired by Freeman (1984) and Orts and Strudler's (2002) research, we regard a stakeholder as any actor who can affect and/or be affected by the activities in question; in our case, policy-making processes influencing the lives of drug users. The reasons for choosing drug user groups as stakeholders as the focus of our analysis are threefold. First, it is important to examine how a relatively new category of stakeholders has entered policy processes which have traditionally been dominated by rather established groups such as politicians, social workers, and medical doctors (Beccaria & Rolando, 2013; Duke et al., 2013; Eisenbach-Stangl, 2013; Frank et al., 2013; Moskalewicz & Welbel, 2013). Second, the emergence of drug user groups as stakeholders brings a new perspective into the policy-making process in the drug field by adding the voices of the citizens who are most affected by the laws and policies. This is not a specific trend for the drug field: the engagement of new user and citizen stakeholder groups has developed rapidly in the last decades in other policy areas related to health, education, housing, criminal justice, and psychiatry (see for example Bjerge et al, 2014; Mol, 2008; Rivera, 2003; Valenta & Berg, 2010). Third, and consequently, user groups as stakeholders have not been the subject of much research scrutiny and there is also a need to try out analytical approaches for studying this particular group of stakeholders as they are not often prominent in the public debate (Anker et al., 2006a). User groups do not have a long tradition of organizing themselves; they often lead unstable lives which complicate formal, long-term organization and participation; and the activities they engage in are sometimes illegal and often socially stigmatized. All these factors make it difficult for people who use drugs to be represented as well as to participate in public debates and policymaking processes.

The idea to explore user groups as stakeholders emerged from an ongoing study with researchers from Austria, Denmark, Italy, and the UK focusing on various stakeholders' roles and influence in the addiction fields. As explained in the Foreword to this volume, the project formed a part of the EU-funded project Addictions and Lifestyles in Contemporary Europe: Reframing Addictions Project (ALICE RAP).[2] Other cases of stakeholders' roles and influence studied in the same project were in opioid substitution treatment policy (Beccaria & Rolando, 2013; Duke et al., 2013; Eisenbach-Stangl, 2013; Frank et al., 2013; Moskalewicz & Welbel, 2013); alcohol policy (Beccaria & Rolando, 2014; Thom et al., 2015); and in drug consumption rooms (Houborg & Frank 2014; Houborg et al., 2014). The case studies are based on documentary and literature analyses as well as individual in-depth interviews with key informants (seventeen interviews each in Austria and Denmark, nineteen in Italy, twenty in the UK). The informants represent a broad range of stakeholders such as treatment providers, policymakers, representatives from scientific societies, advocacy groups, users' organizations, general practitioners, magistrates, and representatives from the pharmaceutical industry. The informants were interviewed about the role and influence of different stakeholders—including user groups—in the development of national drug policies.

Analyses revealed that drug users and drug user groups played rather different roles in the different countries. In some countries user groups were very active and visible, while in others they were almost absent, or at least quite invisible. We also found it difficult to place drug user groups' voices within the existing literature and the analytical frameworks that we employed in these studies, because they are not very sensitive to unconventional stakeholders such as drug users (Kingdon 1984/1995; Sabatier & Jenkins-Smith, 1993, 1999). Researchers from all four countries (the UK, Denmark, Italy, and Austria) therefore decided to conduct a further examination of the data they had collected on user groups as stakeholders in drug policy processes. Additional and complementary data was collected in order to facilitate analysis around this specific focus on user groups.

It was clear that the analysis of user groups as stakeholders called for other theoretical perspectives enabling investigation of the role of user groups.

Previously, social movement organization theories have been employed in analyses of user groups' influence (Anker et al., 2006a; Frank et al., 2012; Tops, 2006). However, user groups can be difficult to understand through this perspective because they are different from more traditional social movements—such as civil rights, labour unions, women's rights, and peace movements—which are less introverted, defensive, and vulnerable than drug user groups (Anker et al., 2006a). Therefore, we decided to explore Backstrand's (2003, 2004) concepts of participation, representation, and democratization as a way to examine the political space that this group of stakeholders take and/or are given. That is, we will apply this approach as an analytical lens rather than a strict scheme for analysis. The chapter sets out to demonstrate *how* and *why* the level of user participation, representation, and involvement in democratization processes varies from country to country. Before presenting the analysis and discussing our findings, we will briefly contextualize the developments and the definitions of drug user groups and outline our analytical approach.

6.2 **Drug user groups: definitions and background**

Drug user groups are primarily groups run by active drug users, who represent drug users and who help and attend to matters concerning drug users (Goossens, 2008). 'Active drug users' are people who either use drugs or are enrolled in substitution treatment. It does not include former drug users. There are different kinds of user groups with different kinds of purposes. A distinction is often made between service user groups, on the one hand, and activist user groups, on the other (Mold & Berridge, 2010; Van Hout & McElrath, 2012). The first kind of user group primarily focuses their activities on influencing the development of treatment services. These groups are most often local and take a point of departure in drug users as clients or social service users. In contrast, activist user groups, besides providing peer support, have wider political, social, and health-related agendas linked to human rights, destigmatization, decriminalization, empowerment, harm reduction, and increased access to healthcare facilities (Mold & Berridge, 2008). These user groups are often larger; they may be regional or even national in scope. In practice, many drug user groups that can be defined as 'activist user groups' focus not only on activist-oriented activities but also on improving treatment service facilities in a similar way as the service user groups, which makes it difficult to clearly distinguish between the two groups (Bjerge et al, in press, 2016; Houborg, 2012). In this chapter we focus on the activist user groups, or the activist aspects of the groups under study.[3]

The first activist user group was established in the 1970s in Holland (Frank et al., 2012; Hunt et al., 2010). In other countries, such as the UK, activist user groups were established in the 1980s, originally emerging from fears of an HIV epidemic among people who inject drugs (Mold & Berridge, 2010; Thom et al., 2013). A variety of activist user groups emerged in the 1990s (Anker et al., 2006a; Hunt et al., 2010; Mold & Berridge, 2010). These range from small-scale, local groups aiming to challenge local conditions to wider national and international networks and associations. In 2005, according to Goossens (2008), there were drug user groups in fourteen European countries, including Denmark, UK, and the Netherlands. Many of these groups have joined the international umbrella organization for drug user groups, INPUD (International Network for People who Use Drugs), established in 2006 at the harm reduction conference in Vancouver (http://www.inpud.net). This network is worldwide and has about sixty drug user groups in its membership. In addition, the International Harm Reduction Association (renamed Harm Reduction International in 2011; http://www.ihra.net) and the European Coalition for Just and Effective Drug Policies (http://www.encod.org) have been important stakeholders contributing to the development of national drug user groups (Hunt et al., 2010). These international networks have become increasingly prominent through their lobbying activities and participation in policy conferences and debates. For example, they have been influential stakeholders in the development of harm reduction initiatives (Hunt et al., 2010), and the INPUD is invited annually to speak and participate in the high level sessions of the Commission for Narcotic Drugs at the United Nations office in Vienna. Nevertheless, activist user groups are often confronted with challenges relating to funding, accreditation, and visible political influence (Frank et al., 2013; Mold & Berridge, 2010).

6.3 **Representation, participation, and democratization**

Certain individuals are powerful stakeholders because they occupy important positions in policy networks, such as government ministers and civil servants. But for many stakeholders, representation is a matter of both abilities and possibilities to engage in collective action. For example, drug users may find it difficult to influence substitution treatment policy unless they are able, in one way or another, to act collectively; for example, by organizing in unions (Anker et al., 2006b; Asmussen, 2003). The study of drug policy making and the influence of user groups as stakeholders can benefit from taking into account the opportunities and constraints to engage in collective action. Different societies provide different opportunities for collective action. In some, procedures for policymaking processes will involve mostly formally recognized institutionalized stakeholders (e.g. organizations, unions). Other societies have a greater number of procedures for ensuring the involvement of noninstitutional stakeholders (i.e. people who are temporarily organized around an issue). By studying the opportunities and limits of collective action, it becomes possible to say something about the stakes or concerns that will be represented in the development of drug policies; by whom and the role that the different actors play.

In line with this thinking, Backstrand's framework for civic science and expertise—especially the concepts of *representation, participation*, and *democratization*—can be adapted as an approach for our analysis to explore if and how user groups are involved in policy processes as well as for exploring the roles and activities of user groups in the development of drug policy, practice, and research (Backstrand, 2003, 2004). 'Civic science' encapsulates 'the various attempts to increase public participation in the production and use of scientific knowledge' (Backstrand, 2003, p. 24). A key theme in the ALICE RAP case studies of stakeholders is how they both use and produce knowledge and evidence. When looking at drug policy governance, key questions include 'what counts as expertise?', 'what counts as evidence?', and 'who decides what counts?' (Duke & Thom, 2014). Drug users can be viewed as 'experts' through experience; their forms of knowledge and evidence (e.g. experiential, tacit and embodied knowledges) can be employed in drug policy debates. Backstrand (2003, 2004) argues that there is a constant re-evaluation of the status of expert knowledge and the boundaries between scientific and nonscientific knowledge, expert and lay knowledge, global and local knowledge, and risk assessment and risk management. In Backstrand's framework, efforts are made by scientists to reach a wider group of stakeholders (including the public), to communicate scientific results more widely, and to help contribute to developing scientific literacy. The framework emphasizes a bottom-up approach characterized by public deliberation, communication, and participation which challenges the traditional top-down approaches led by experts who have been given privileged status. Civic expertise recognizes the plurality of expert knowledge and includes informal expertise (i.e. experiential, local, tacit, and indigenous) as valid expertise and/or knowledge (Karvonen & Brand, 2014).

Civic science is underpinned by three different but interconnected dimensions: representation, participation, and democratization (Backstrand, 2003, 2004). Although Backstrand applies these dimensions specifically to the development of civic science, they can also be usefully employed in a more general sense to explore user involvement in drug policy debates and development. For example, *participation* could refer to attempts to increase 'public' participation by bringing a wider range of stakeholders into policymaking processes. In particular, the extent of participation of users and user groups could be examined as well as various techniques employed to increase participation. Examples of this might include user groups connected with research studies, consultation exercises, user forums, and membership on advisory and steering groups for research and policy initiatives.

Representation could refer to attempts to reverse the skewed representation in policy development and the narrow group of people who are viewed as 'experts'. This involves incorporating multiple stakeholders in the policymaking process and recognizing the 'expertise' of other groups, including users. A key question is how far have different user groups been involved in developing 'knowledge' and policy in relation to drug issues, where user groups refers to women, indigenous people, users or clients of different types of services, and stakeholders at various levels (local, national, and international). Knowledge transmission is often focused on the national and international levels, which may omit important knowledge, expertise, and experience occurring at local levels. As Stone (2012, p. 7) argues, '[P]ractitioner insights, grassroots knowledge and communal voices do not have the same credence or value as 'expert' deliberations' (p. 7). This means that inequalities between different forms of knowledge/evidence and experts/actors are produced and reproduced.

The final dimension within Backstrand's framework is the process of *democratization*, or how far institutions involved in policy making incorporate democratic principles into their work to include the voices of users and collaborate with user groups. Civic expertise involves participatory models of specialized knowledge. As Karvonen and Brand (2014) argue, this involves the development of democratic processes where experts and non-experts work together as collaborators. However, such an 'arrangement does not guarantee an equitable distribution of power between stakeholders but, at the very least, allows for the possibility that non-experts voices can be heard' (Karvonen & Brand, 2014, p. 225).

Drawing on Backstrand's approach and the interconnected dimensions of representation, participation, and democratization, we will now account for the main trends in participation and representation in the UK, Denmark, Italy, and Austria. Subsequently, we will synthesize the analysis by discussing democratization processes and the inclusion of 'non-experts' as recognized actors in how drug-related issues are managed in the four countries. It will become evident that the four countries have very different traditions for handling the issue of users as stakeholders. The UK and Denmark have actively engaged users in policy development for the past decades, whereas Italy and Austria do not have established mechanisms for involving users.

6.4 Participation and representation in the UK, Denmark, Austria, and Italy

6.4.1 The UK

During the late 1980s, the number of stakeholders involved in British drug policy issues increased to encompass a more diversified range of groups, including voluntary agencies, general practitioners, and drug users themselves. The increase in heroin users and the HIV crisis provided a window of opportunity for different stakeholders to influence the direction of policy and practice. A more multidisciplinary approach to the drug problem emerged with an increased range of services offered to drug users through the Central Funding Initiative (MacGregor et al., 1991). As Mold and Berridge (2008, p. 455) argue, this signalled a shift away from the medical response to drug use that had operated since the 1960s and permitted the voices of other stakeholders to be heard.

During this phase, there was increasing participation and representation of users as they became more visible and active in drug policy debates. Drug user groups formed at the local level—such as the Merseyside Drug Users Group in Liverpool, the Nottingham Drug Dependents Anonymous, and Mainline in Manchester—grew in strength and were successful in their lobbying efforts regarding the development of harm reduction initiatives (e.g. increased methadone prescribing and needle exchange provision). During the 1990s, people who used drugs began to organize in the UK into a politically active user movement which agitated for drug policy and practice reform as well as contributed to the development and delivery of services at local and national levels (Mold & Berridge, 2008). There were user groups involved in state sponsored user involvement concerned mainly with service development and those involved in campaigning for drug users, such as the UK Harm Reduction Alliance (a coalition of drug users and health, social care and criminal justice workers that aim to place public health and human rights at the centre of service provision for drug users), Transform (a charitable think tank that campaigns for the legal regulation of drugs), and Release (a charity that provides free advice and information on drug use and legal issues and campaigns for drug law reform).

The activities by user groups involved in the development of services were aided by a number of wider initiatives (including the Citizen's Charter and the *Health and Social Care Act 2001*), which aimed to involve the patient or service user in care and treatment decisions (Mold & Berridge, 2008). A new user-led group, the Alliance (originally known as the Methadone Alliance) emerged in 1999. Its aims were to improve the quality and availability of treatment and to facilitate the voices of users in treatment and in the development of national and international drug policy.

With the establishment of the National Treatment Agency (NTA) and increased funding for treatment in 2001, there were various initiatives for greater user involvement in the development of drug policy, practice, and research. A user representative was appointed on the NTA board and users were represented at regional and local levels in service planning and delivery. For example, Drug Action Teams, which are responsible for drug issues at the local level, include users in the decision making around service provision. In 2003, the NTA set up the Experts by Experience programme which aimed to equip users with practical skills to enable them to actively participate in debates on drug policy and practice and advocate changes in treatment provision.

Lay and experiential knowledge also began to be viewed as important in the deliberations of expert committees around drug issues. For example, a wide range of stakeholders provided evidence to the House of Commons Home Affairs Committee inquiry into drug policy. In addition to traditional medical 'experts', advocacy and activist groups, think tanks, treatment providers, academics, pharmaceutical companies, user groups, and users representing themselves were heard. An example of the latter was celebrity comedian, Russell Brand, who provided evidence in person as a key witness (Home Affairs Committee, 2012). This indicates a broadening of the traditional concepts of 'expert' and 'stakeholder', and can be viewed as an attempt to increase both representation and participation of drug users in the policy arena.

Research on stakeholders in the recent recovery debates in the UK found that more inclusive approaches, such as consultations and representation on expert committees, have given opportunities for new voices to be heard, including the ones of user groups (some of which advocate abstinence-based recovery), and consequently for them to exert some influence over the dialogue surrounding drug treatment policy (Duke et al., 2013; Duke & Thom, 2014). However, it is interesting to note that when methadone maintenance treatment (MMT) was being questioned from 2005 onwards, there appeared to be no public defence of it by many of the traditional user groups which had advocated for its expansion in the late 1980s and 1990s. Some stakeholders argued that service user and user activist groups advocating harm reduction had become complacent and failed to recognize the strength of the growing abstinence-based recovery movement, and that the role of methadone in treatment provision could be questioned or displaced (Duke et al., 2013). With the confidence that harm reduction and MMT had become successfully embedded in the treatment infrastructure in Britain, some stakeholders argued that the harm reduction movement had turned away from national and local debates and become increasingly focused on international issues. With the shift towards a 'recovery'-oriented drug strategy, there were still debates around the future role of opioid substitution treatment within this framework.

In order to settle the debates, the NTA set up an expert group to examine the evidence base for different types of substitute prescribing. The expert group had representatives from a diverse range of backgrounds, including user groups. However, as some of the stakeholders indicated in the interviews of this study, the degree of 'real' participation was questionable (Duke & Thom, 2014). Some felt that the expert committee was dominated by 'doctors' and those with 'traditional expertise', rather than the representatives with lay and experiential knowledge.

6.4.2 Denmark

In contrast to the UK, the voices of users as active stakeholders in Denmark have mainly been represented by one Copenhagen-based user group, the Danish Drug Users Union (DDUU).[4] It was established in 1993 by drug users enrolled in a methadone treatment institution (Anker, 2006). In 1995 the DDUU was invited to have a representative on the Narcotics Council under the Ministry of Social Affairs, an advisory body to the then Social Democratic–led government. This board discussed drug policy and published several reports dealing with the administration of MMT, the implementation of harm reduction measures, as well as what harm reduction measures were needed (Frank et al., 2013). While the board did not have direct political power, it was viewed as a type of think tank providing knowledge and evidence for new lines of development in drug policy (Houborg, 2012). Many of these suggestions for policy development—especially the introduction of harm reduction measures—were seen as too liberal by some of the political parties at the time. Liberals and conservatives in Denmark were not keen on the recommendations emerging from the board. In 2002, when a new liberal/conservative government came to power, the board was terminated. It was replaced by a broader board of 'socially excluded citizens', including homeless people, people with mental health problems, sex workers, and citizens living below the poverty line. The DDUU did not manage to get a representative on to this board and lost their position as active participants on this political platform (Frank et al., 2013). In that sense, the possibilities of drug users participating in Danish policy processes at the national level can best be defined as rather unstable, depending on shifting governmental priorities.

Although deprived of a voice on government advisory boards, drug users' voices are represented in other ways in policy processes. Their voices have been strengthened by alliances with other stakeholders in the drug policy field, and through informal alliances with the NGO Street Lawyer (established in 2001) and with a leading physician in Copenhagen, Peter Ege, who has long been a prominent voice in the field. Drug users have managed to remain represented in the political debates. For example, a stakeholder from the DDUU described how the alliance with The Street Lawyer led to a change in practice whereby liquid methadone was no longer mixed with juice at treatment centres (Frank et al., 2013). The practice of mixing methadone with juice was undertaken in order to ensure that users did not inject the methadone. Despite this precautionary practice, users continued to inject the mixture which could cause physical injuries such as infections and sores that, in more severe cases, could develop into semi chronic conditions/endocarditis due to the presence of the juice.

Further evidence of the representation and participation of drug users in the drug policy developments is that the DDUU is occasionally invited to comment on hearing statements before policy recommendations are sent out by the Ministry of Health or the Ministry of Social Affairs. For example, together with eighty-two other groups, in 2013 the DDUU was invited to comment on recommendations on the prevention of drug use (*forebyggelsespakke*) from the National Board of Health to the ninety-eight municipalities in Denmark; the DDUU was on the list of groups to comment on the draft for the revision of the *Act on Euphoria-Inducing Drugs* to implement safe injection sites in Denmark (Houborg & Frank, 2014); and in 2012 the DDUU was invited to comment on the draft for the EU's new drug strategy. In this sense, the DDUU has become a legitimate voice and recognized as a relevant stakeholder to consult in policy matters related to drug issues.

More indirectly, the voices of Danish drug users started to become increasingly heard in policy processes elsewhere in the 1990s; for example, when new legislation on social services came into being (Socialministeriet, 1998). This legislation made it mandatory to include citizens in the delivery and implementation of different kinds of social services, on both an individual and organizational level (Bjerge et al, 2014; Frank & Bjerge, 2011). For example, social service institutions were now obliged to write up action plans and involve users more actively in the treatment provided. Thus users of welfare services participate in the development of service delivery, as well as, increasingly, recognized as legitimate voices or 'experts' in the field through the DDUU.

6.4.3 **Italy**

Contrary to the UK and Denmark, the participation and representation of drug users in drugs policy is less visible in Italy and practically nonexistent in Austria. An Italian study of drug policy stakeholders demonstrated the very low influence of drug user groups in the development of Italian drug policy (Beccaria & Rolando, 2013). For example, of the seventy members making up the national consulting board of the Anti-drugs Policies Department that last gathered in 2009, there were no representatives from specific drug user groups. Even though there are no examples of proper 'activist user groups' at national level, at local level somewhere there are 'service user groups' (Mold & Berridge, 2010; Van Hout & McElrath, 2012) whose action—often stimulated by and carried out in close cooperation with service providers—is primarily aimed at improving the treatment service and at facilitating the engagement of new patients.

The situation was more animated during the 1990s when the Italian debate on drug treatment was at its peak, mainly due to the challenges of the HIV epidemic. As well as in the UK and Denmark, the crisis provided a window of opportunity for the development of MMT (Frank et al., 2013; Thom et al., 2013), but in Italy the catholic church influence made this process particularly difficult. Prior to this, heroin addiction was treated primarily in therapeutic communities (TC)—often led by religious leaders—using educational and/or psychosocial methods. Opioid substitution treatment was hindered by the church's position, which was that the only solution to addiction was total abstinence from all drugs (legal and illegal); harm reduction approaches were considered an avoidance of personal responsibility. This position was exploited by the right-wing politicians and supported by the TCs as well as by groups of parents and by other users' relatives, such as spouses. In fact, at the time, parents' groups were more organized and visible than user groups.

As noted previously, in the early 1990s, mainly due to the alarming situation caused by the HIV epidemic among drug users, Italian drug policy debate was reopened. A number of stakeholders, primarily the public addiction services supported by researchers, took the opportunity to influence the policy debate on substitution treatment. This would eventually lead to a possibility for the establishment of local substitution treatment (Beccaria & Rolando, 2013). Furthermore, during that period an informal movement emerged that tried to complete a reform to abolish the penalization of personal drug use.

In 1996 a charter of drug consumers' rights was presented publicly in Florence by an aggregation of different stakeholders, including user groups. The users were mainly heroin users claiming the right to be treated and to choose the most appropriate type of treatment. The charter was presented again in 1997 during the second governmental conference on drugs held in Naples. However, according to stakeholders, the charter did not have great political resonance and did not immediately affect treatment provision. Changes on such a structural level would take a longer time and were primarily the outcome of an internal debate in the treatment services sector (Beccaria & Rolando, 2013). In other words, user groups did not succeed in influencing policy processes and debates at the national level; their influence remained mainly limited to the local level, as service user groups.

In 2010, after a long period of inactivity, new stakeholders have appeared in the Italian debate on drug use. This could indicate a shift towards a new political debate, one that includes the drug users' perspective. During a national meeting organized by the Italian Network for Harm Reduction (ITARDD) in 2014, focusing on drug users and their role as peers in treatment, a new charter of rights was presented. This new charter is different from the rather one-dimensional focus on rights to treatment in the 1996 charter. Instead, emphasis is placed on the right to consume and the right not to be stigmatized and sanctioned because of drug use. Furthermore, the document has been signed by different associations, both movements active at the national level and on wider issues—such as the ITARDD and the League for the Fight Against AIDS (LILA)—and by local user groups.

Besides the older generation of heroin users linked to treatment services, the 2014 meeting was attended by a new generation of users, including cannabis users promoting social clubs, representatives of social centres, and rave goers. A representative of the European Coalition for Just and Effective Drug Policies commented that the presence of different generations and types of Italian drug consumers was unusual compared to other countries.

Nevertheless, the process of promoting and circulating the charter has just begun; the degree to which it spreads will depend mainly on the initiative of local groups that present it to services and municipalities at the local level. However, it has also been circulated on the Internet, thus potentially stimulating a wider public debate. It is possible that new types of less stigmatized user groups and increased use of the social media will enable Italian users to participate more actively as stakeholders in the current drug policy processes.

6.4.4 **Austria**

In Austria, drug users never became key stakeholders in drug policy. Although supported by drug professionals, all user organizations established during the 1970s and 1980s, mainly in Vienna, were weak and short-lived. Most were service user groups, such as the Association of Former Drug Addicts, the first drug clinic in the late 1970s, which employed ex-users as therapists. The association dissolved after a few years without having realized its modest aim: to organize aftercare for the clients of the clinic. In the 1980s a user organization campaigned for substitution treatment, and another tried to help formers users set up in business after treatment. Not even the change of the treatment paradigm from abstinence to harm reduction in the mid-1980s and the establishment of low-threshold facilities and a substitution programme—which in many countries created an opportunity for the development of user organizations—led to an increase in user groups in Austria.

Also short-lived and without remarkable impact on drug policy were the occasional initiatives of users to legalize cannabis (e.g. INHALE in the 1980s; Eisenbach-Stangl et al., 2008). Only self-help organizations of relatives of drug users, mainly mothers, were somewhat more numerous, longer-lived, spread out geographically, and effective: they provided information and advice to parents of users, and in one case established an innovative outpatient drug service. These self-help groups of relatives disbanded during the 1990s, replaced by professionally guided groups for relatives (Kranzl, 2006).

The poor organization of users is indicative of their distance from, and even lack of interest in, political issues around drugs. One drug professional interviewed for the case study recalled that drug clients thought she and her colleagues were 'mad' to campaign for heroin as a substitution substance during the 1980s. Lack of interest in drug policy might have been promoted by the historically early and comprehensive medicalization of drug use and drug users (Zobel, 2014), which provided diversified welfare and care for users, but which also turned them into individualized, passive, and dependent clients. The strength of medicalization in Austria is indicated by a high coverage of problem users by drug services and by the substitution programmes. Moreover, therapeutic measures are favoured over penal and legal responses (in Austria only 7 per cent of all drug offenders are fined or imprisoned; Bericht, 2014). Thus users are kept 'busy with medicalization'—as another interviewee suggests—and beyond that, with the time-consuming management of everyday life: with social and health problems and the organization of needed welfare measures, whose availability is made difficult by bureaucratic barriers (Eisenbach-Stangl & Spirig, 2010).

Users' lack of interest in drug policy in Austria is not the only factor explaining the missing public voice of users. It is paralleled by the political system's lack of interest, which never encouraged users' activities, but did listen to their advocates—the drug professionals (i.e. the multiprofessional members of the staff of the extended and diversified drug services and drug administration, continuously increasing in numbers since the 1970s).

To summarize this part of the study, we have four very different cases of representation and participation in the countries under study. In the next section, we will discuss the democratization aspects of the cases.

6.5 **Democratization**

By exploring the participation and representation of user groups in the UK, Denmark, Italy, and Austria, it has become evident that the inclusion of drug users as stakeholders in policy processes varies. In the framework of Backstrand (2003, 2004), the extent to which these 'non-expert' voices are heard and given opportunity to challenge established power relations is related to how far policymaking institutions have incorporated democratic principles in their work (cf. Karvonen & Brand, 2014). The different ways in which such principles have been incorporated in the countries discussed can be linked to different factors in the specific countries. Different democratic challenges need to be overcome if users are to be active stakeholders in policy processes.

6.5.1 The UK

Britain has been active in integrating the expertise and knowledge of a wider group of stakeholders, including drug users, into policymaking processes. Since the 1980s, there has been increased representation and participation of drug users in policy structures at national, regional, and local levels. The development of user groups was aided by the impact of HIV and the need to develop harm reduction techniques. As in the Danish case, their activities have been facilitated further by wider transformations in health and social services, which emphasize user involvement and the rights of patients and consumers in service provision. The HIV issue provided an opportunity for collaboration and partnership between user groups and the more 'traditional' expert groups.

However, this does not mean that their representation and participation in these debates have been unified or necessarily strong and powerful. There have been conflicts between different representatives depending on their ideologies and ambitions (Mold & Berridge, 2008). Recent developments in British drug policy have rekindled divisions within the drug field between harm reductionists and those who advocate abstinence-based recovery. This has been mirrored in the different groups representing users and 'recovering' users. Different user groups with varying goals, perspectives, and tacit knowledge are competing against one another to be heard within policy spaces. Recent governmental committees and the various mechanisms for user participation, such as consensus committees, have ensured the representation and participation of user groups with different perspectives. However, visibility and participation do not necessarily translate into impact, power, and influence. It is unclear whether these different forms of tacit knowledge are given the same value as the traditional 'expert' knowledge in policy deliberations.

6.5.2 Denmark

Denmark has also been active in integrating knowledge and expertise of drug users in policy processes, although the actual outcome can be difficult to pinpoint, with the exception of some of the examples presented earlier in this chapter. The universalistic Nordic welfare regime has traditionally aimed for inclusion of marginalized groups in the public system (Esping-Andersen 1990), and perhaps therefore the idea of including drug users as experts in policy processes has been easier to implement in Denmark. Further, the emergence and manifestation of user groups as stakeholders can be linked to a coinciding of different interests. For example, in the 1990s and onwards, research points to more general societal trends in which Danish politicians and NGOs have challenged social workers' expert positions (Bjerge, 2012; Bjerge & Nielsen, 2014; Frank et al., 2013). As a result, treatment providers, for example, are to be facilitators of users' wishes and needs rather than experts in how users should lead their lives (Asmussen, 2003; Bjerge, 2008, 2009; Houborg & Bjerge, 2011).

Such respect for clients' lived expertise does not apply only to the drug field, but also to all other social and health services (Bjerregaard, 2007; Johanson, 2007; Torfing, 1999; Villadsen, 2008; Vohnsen, 2011). Thus, there has been an articulated public policy agenda characterized by more focus on the rights of users, more individual freedom, and more self-management by users. However, the Danish case also highlights that users' voices on the agenda may currently be minimized because of the lack of direct political participation. Furthermore, a stakeholder interviewed for the study notes that some of the critique that was raised in the 1990s and 2000s by users and their representatives has now been transformed into bureaucratic auditing and control measures—via user evaluations or local users' forums—rather than into restructuring organizations and services (Frank et al., 2013). In that sense, incorporating users' participation and representation in the political and welfare service agenda might, in some respects, have silenced the criticism and transformed it into new ways of trying to steer and manage the citizens in question (for further discussion, see Cruikshank, 1999; Frank & Bjerge, 2011; Villadsen, 2008).

6.5.3 **Italy**

In Italy, the lack of drug user groups as policy stakeholders is mainly perceived by representatives in the field as a symptom of a persistent stigmatization of drug users (Beccaria & Rolando, 2013). Due to this deep-seated stigmatization, drug users have tended to remain hidden and have not been willing to reveal their identity by engagement in drug user activism. Further, the lack of active drug user groups can be related to the decrease in young people's engagement in politics (e.g. through youth councils), which, according to one stakeholder, could be seen as part of a general Italian societal, democratic problem concerning a lack of action aimed at obtaining or defending social rights and participation (Beccaria & Rolando, 2013).

However, examining other kinds of associations, Italy is a lively country with many active client and consumer associations; for example, associations for different kinds of patients (e.g. the national league for the fight against AIDS, and the Italian Association of Alzheimer Disease). Therefore, the stigma explanation seems to be the most credible.

The weight of the stigma on drug users has deep roots in Italian culture. It relates to the fact that under the influence of the Catholic church, drug use has been highly moralized. Indeed, the conceptualization of drug addiction as a disease has never been fully accepted, either by the Catholic church or by the Radicals, the anti-prohibitionist political party. Catholics were afraid that this concept would remove the individual's responsibility for drug use, and the Radicals thought that the disease model would transform users into passive subjects (Beccaria & Rolando, 2014).

The stigmatization of drug users has been further strengthened by the Italian mass media (Beccaria & Rolando, 2014), and is observable even among general practitioners and social workers (Hellman et al., 2014). The institutions involved in policy making have not yet been able to include the voices of drug users directly—only indirectly and partially, through the voices of other kinds of more 'powerful' and less stigmatized stakeholders, such as representatives of the national league for the fight against AIDS (LILA). In that sense, Italy faces democratic challenges in drug policies if drug users' voices are to be included. To do so, it must overcome the persistent moral view and stigmatization of drug use. Currently, however, this seems to be a real possibility because of the changed prevalence and profiles of drug users. Today cannabis users are more numerous, more active, and much less stigmatized than the old heroin users.

6.5.4 **Austria**

In Austria there is no tradition of users' voices in policy processes or the public debate. Users do not articulate their interests in public and in political forums, but their needs and requests are brought forward by active advocates—mainly medical doctors, social workers, and lawyers—who, since the late 1970s, have been acknowledged as 'experts' in drug questions. When drug users participate in research studies, they express alienation towards drug policy but astonishingly high satisfaction with their advocates and the drug services—especially those aimed at harm reduction (e.g. Eisenbach-Stangl et al., 2012). Thus lacking representation and participation of users is to be explained not only by alienation from drug policy but also by their satisfaction with their advocates' activities.

With regard to the partly successful advocacy, it is important to mention that Austrian society to a high degree is penetrated by the political system via compulsory or organized stakeholder groups (in the Austrian case, better labelled as 'traditional interest groups'), which structures all responses to social issues politically and guarantees attention to the needs of their members. Marginalized groups, prominently among them addicts, traditionally are linked to the Social Democratic Party. Consequently, since the 1970s Austrian drug policy and drug services have been determined by interest groups belonging or linked to the party. Prominent among these are drug professionals with close ties to the users. Though advocacy is a conservative way to respond to the needs of marginalized groups—and is probably restricted to traditional societies— according to users and other stakeholders, it was and still is effective in meeting the basic needs of Austrian drug users.

6.6 **Conclusions**

This chapter shows how drug user groups as stakeholders and in policy processes vary significantly in the four countries. Although the examples stem only from four countries, we hope that our findings will stimulate further discussion of the role of users as stakeholders in other European countries as well as worldwide. The discussion will have both democratic and epistemological aspects. The democratic question is whose interests and concerns get to be represented in policy processes; who has the opportunity to participate in such processes? The epistemological question is which kinds of knowledge and experiences are regarded as relevant and allowed to influence how society manages drug-related issues? To explore such important questions, the chapter has taken as its point of departure Backstrand's three concepts of representation, participation, and democratization. Attention has been paid to the fact that user groups and user voices for various reasons are often not very well organized or prominent in public debates, but nevertheless—at times—can play important roles in policy processes.

Overall, the chapter illustrates that the countries represented are only beginning to grapple with the issues of representation, participation, and democratization—apart from Austria, where the process of involving drugs users as experts in policy development has not even begun, but where users seem to be quite satisfied with the way things are. Even within countries such as the UK and Denmark, where these processes have been developed the most, there are limited 'windows' for these processes to emerge and develop. As Backstrand (2004, p. 709) notes, representation and participation do not necessarily lead to democratization or democratic governance. These attempts at greater public participation could be merely 'cosmetic adjustments' which do not challenge the traditional policymaking structures and procedures. Within this model of governance, drug users become 'expert patients' and their knowledge and expertise are tapped into by policymakers. Although this encourages greater representation, participation, and the illusion of 'partnership', it is important to continue to explore the relations of power; for example, between user groups, service providers, and policymakers.

In fact, Zibbell (2004) suggests that in order for drug users to become active participants, the inherent structural inequality underpinning policymaking structures in many European countries need to be contested and challenged altogether. As suggested by the Italian case, perhaps the use of social media such as Twitter, Facebook, self-help sites, and user forums could provide a way for user groups to recruit more widely and transform the ways in which they operate in terms of communicating and organizing—and thereby challenge existing hierarchies of knowledge and influence. Moreover, continuing empirical research on the subject, as well as analytical exploration of user groups as stakeholders, will hopefully shed light on drug users as a particular type of stakeholder possessing important knowledge of how societies can better understand and respond to drug-related issues.

Notes

1 The term 'drug user' is a contested concept. For example, the International Network of People who Use Drugs (INPUD) prefers the term 'people who use drugs', as 'drug user' is seen to reduce the complexity of individuals to one aspect of their lives. For a more detailed discussion, see the statement and position of INPUD on language, identity, inclusivity, and discrimination in the drugs field. http://www.inpud.net/INPUD_Statement_Position_Paper_on_Language_Identity_Inclusivity_Discrimination_Nov2011.pdf

2 Six countries formed part of the work package focusing on stakeholder analyses: Austria, Denmark, Finland, Italy, Poland, and the UK.

3 For further information on service user groups, see Bryant et al. (2008), Fischer et al. (2007), Frank and Bjerge (2011), and Bjerge, Brown, and Davis (forthcoming). This literature shows how service user groups for different reasons have gained more and more ground in influencing the development of treatment provision. Professionals in treatment organizations are encouraged to engage in equal dialogue with users, but are also encouraged, and in some cases required, to include different kinds of tools to enhance the perspectives of service users by setting up user councils, joint meetings, user evaluations, user-driven cafés, etc.

4 Contrary to several other countries (for example, the Netherlands), active drug users in Denmark have only been successful in establishing the DDUU in Copenhagen. While there were attempts to create such a union in Aarhus, the second-biggest city in Denmark, the organization called 'Stris' was practically run by only one man; it has primarily been active as an organization that treatment services in Aarhus could consult to implement user participation at an organizational level (Frank et al., 2012).

References

Anker, J. (2006). Active drug users—struggling for rights and recognition. In J. Anker et al. (Eds.), Drug users and spaces for legitimate action. Helsinki: NAD (Nordic Council for Alcohol and Drug Research). 37–60.

Anker, J., Asmussen, V., Kouvonen, P., & Tops, D. (2006a). Introduction. In J. Anker et al. (Eds.), Drug users and spaces for legitimate action. Helsinki: NAD (Nordic Council for Alcohol and Drug Research). 5–22.

Anker, J., Asmussen, V., Kouvonen, P., & Tops, D. (Eds.). (2006b). Drug users and spaces for legitimate action. Helsinki: Nordic Council for Alcohol and Drug Research (NAD).

Asmussen, V. (2003). User participation: possibilities and limitations on Danish social services directed towards drug users. In E.H. Pedersen & C. Tigerstedt (Eds.), Regulating drugs—between users, the police and social workers. Helsinki: Nordic Council for Alcohol and Drug Research. 11–32.

Backstrand, K. (2003). Civic science for sustainability: reframing the role of experts, policy-makers and citizens in environmental governance. *Global Environmental Politics*, **3**(4), 24–41.

Backstrand, K. (2004). Scientisation vs civic expertise in environmental governance: eco-feminist, eco-modern and post-modern responses. *Environmental Politics*, **13**(4), 695–714.

Beccaria, F., & Rolando, S. (2013). Stakeholders' role in contemporary 'substitute drug' prescribing policies in Italy. *Substance Use & Misuse*, **48**(11), 943–953.

Beccaria F., & Rolando S. (2014). The Italian politics of alcohol: the creation of a public arena at the end of the 20th century. *International Journal of Drug Policy*, **26**(7) 662–69.

Beccaria F., Rolando S., Hellman M., Bujalski M., & Lemmens P. (2014). From criminals to celebrities: perceptions of 'the addict' in the print press from four European countries. *Substance Use & Misuse* **50**(4), 439–453.

Bericht. (2014). Bericht zur Drogensituation 2014 im Auftrag der Europäischen Beobachtungsstelle für Drogen und Drogensucht und des Bundesministeriums für Gesundheit (Report on the drug situation 2014 on behalf of the European Monitoring Centre for Drugs and Drug Addiction and the Federal Ministry for Health Affairs), Wien: Gesundheit Österreich & Bundesministerium für Gesundheit.

Bjerge, B. (2008). The re-organization of drug treatment in Denmark—a welfare reform as policy. In V. Asmussen Frank et al. (Eds.), Drug policy—history, theory, and consequences: examples from Denmark and USA. Åarhus: Aarhus University Press. 209–232.

Bjerge, B. (2009). Mellem vision og praksis: strukturreformen, rusmiddelbureaukrati og [New public management]. Copenhagen: University of Copenhagen, Institute of Sociology.

Bjerge, B. (2012). Structural reform as New Public Management policy. Three dilemmas in Danish substance misuse treatment In M. Hellman et al. (Eds.), A welfare policy patchwork—negotiating the public good in times of transition. Stockholm: NVC. 181–201.

Bjerge, B., Brown, C., & Davis, G. (in press, 2016). User perspectives. In: Kolind, T., Thom, B. and Hunt, G. (eds) Handbook on drug and alcohol studies. Thousand Oaks, CA: Sage.

Bjerge, B., & Nielsen, B. (2014). Empowered and self-managing users in methadone treatment? *European Journal of Social Work*, **17**(1), 74–87.

Bjerge, B., Nielsen, B., & Frank, V.A. (2014). Rationalities of choice and practicalities of care. *Contemporary Drug Problems*, **41**, 57–90.

Bjerregaard, T. (2007). Brugerinddragelse og faglighed i socialpsykiatrien. In B. Bjerge & B. Selmer (Eds.), Det sociale arbejdes daglige praksis. Perspektiver på brugerinddragelse og retssikkerhed Aarhus: Aarhus Universitetsforlag, 57–74.

Bryant, J., Saxton, M., Madden, A., Bath, N., & Robinson, S. (2008). Consumer participation in the planning and delivery of drug treatment services: the current arrangements. *Drug and Alcohol Review*, **27**(2), 130–137.

Carta dei diritti delle persone che usano sostanze [Charter of drug users' rights]. (2014). Genova. http://www.sostanze.info/articolo/carta-dei-diritti-delle-persone-che-usano-sostanze

Cruikshank, B. (1999). The will to empower. Ithaca, NY: Cornell University Press.

Duke, K., Herring, R., Thickett, A., & Thom, B. (2013). Substitution treatment in the era of 'recovery': an analysis of stakeholder roles and policy windows in Britain. *Substance Use & Misuse*, **48**, 966–976.

Duke, K. & Thom, B. (2014) The role of evidence and the expert in contemporary processes of governance: the case of opioid substitution treatment policy in England. *International Journal of Drug Policy*, **25**, 964–971.

Eisenbach-Stangl, I. (2013). Deviance or innovation? Recent changes of drug substitution treatment in policy in Austria. *Substance Use & Misuse*, **48**, 1010–1021.

Eisenbach-Stangl, I., Pilgram, A., & Reidl, C. (2008). Wiener Drogenpolitik 1970–2005. Außen- und Innenansichten. Occasional publication series of the European Centre for Social Welfare Policy and Research, Wien.

Eisenbach-Stangl, I., Reidl, C. & G. Schmied (2012). Notquartier und Spritzentausch. Die Wiener Drogenszene im Gespräch. Münster: Lit-Verlag.

Eisenbach-Stangl, I. & H. Spirig (2010). Auch Drogenabhängige werden alter . . . Zur Lebenssituation einer Randgruppe. Occasional publication series, Vienna: European Centre for Welfare Policy and Research.

Esping-Andersen, G. (1990). The three worlds of welfare capitalism. Cambridge: Polity Press.

Fischer, J., Jenkins, N., Bloor, M., Neale, J., & Berney, L. (2007). Drug user involvement in treatment decisions. York: Joseph Rowntree Foundation.

Frank, V.A., Anker, J., & Tammi, T. (2012). Drug user organizations in the Nordic countries—local, national, and international dimensions. *Substance Use & Misuse*, **47**, 462–473.

Frank, V.A., & Bjerge, B. (2011). Empowerment in drug treatment: dilemmas in implementing policy in welfare institutions. *Social Sciences & Medicine*, **73**, 201–208.

Frank, V. A., Bjerge, B., & Houborg, E. (2013). Shifts in opioid substitution treatment policy in Denmark from 2000–2011. *Substance Use & Misuse*, **48**, 997–1009.

Freeman, R.E. (1984). Strategic management: a stakeholder approach. Boston, MA: Pitman.

Goossens, S. (2008). Drug user activism—an overview. In G. Bröring & E. Schatz (Eds.), Empowerment and self-organisations of drug users: experiences and lessons learned. Amsterdam: Foundation Regenboog AMOC. 117–133.

Hellman, M., Majamäki, M., Beccaria, F., Egerer, M., Rolando, S., Bujalski, M.,& Moskalewicz, J. (2014). Professional images of addiction. ALICE RAP Deliverable 3.2, Work Package 3. http://www.alicerap.eu/about-alice-rap/areas-a-workpackages/area-1-ownership-of-addiction.html

Home Affairs Committee (2012) Drugs: breaking the cycle. Ninth report of session 2012–13. London: Stationery Office Ltd.

Houborg, E. (2012). The political pharmacology of methadone and heroin in Danish drug policy. *Contemporary Drug Problems*, **39**(Spring), 155–192.

Houborg, E. & Bjerge, B. (2011). Drug policy, control & welfare. *Drugs: Education, Prevention and Policy*, **18**(1), 16–231.

Houborg, E. & Frank, V.A. (2014). Drug consumption rooms and the role of politics and governance in policy processes. *International Journal of Drug Policy*, **25**(5), 972–977.

Houborg, E., Frank, V.A., & Bjerge, B. (2014). From zero-tolerance to non-enforcement: Creating a new space for drug policing in Copenhagen, Denmark. *Contemporary Drug Problems*, **41**(2), 261–291.

Hunt, N., Albert, E., & Sánchez, V.M. (2010). User involvement and user organizing in harm reduction. In T. Rhode & D. Hedrich (Eds.), Harm reduction: evidence, impacts and challenges. Luxembourg: European Monitoring Centre for Drugs and Drug Addiction. 333–354.

Johanson, M.E. (2007). Med lidelser i fokus. Empowerment på et rehabiliteringscenter for traumatiserede flygtninge. In B. Bjerge & B. Selmer (Eds.), Det sociale arbejdes daglige praksis. Perspektiver på brugerinddragelse og retssikkerhed. Aarhus: Aarhus University Press. 95–114

Karvonen, A., & Brand, R. (2014). Expertise: specialized knowledge in environmental politics and sustainability. In P.G. Harris (Ed.), Routledge handbook of global environmental politics. London: Routledge. 215–230.

Kingdon, J. (1995). Agendas, alternatives and public policies (2nd ed.). Boston: Little Brown. (1st ed. 1984)

Kranzl, V. (2006). Selbsthilfegruppen für Eltern Drogensüchtiger und ihre zivilgesellschaftlichen Aktivitäten Diplomarbeit an der Fakultät für Sozialwissenschaften an der Universität Wien.

MacGregor, S., Ettorre, B., Coomber, R., Crosier, A., & Lodge, H. (1991). Drug services in England and the impact of the Central Funding Initiative. London: ISDD.

Mol, A. (2008). Health and the problem of patient choice. London: Routledge.

Mold, A., & Berridge, V. (2008). 'The rise of the user'? voluntary organizations, the state and illegal drugs in England since the 1960s. *Drugs: Education, Prevention and Policy*, **15**(5), 451–461.

Mold, A., & Berridge, V. (2010). Voluntary action and illegal drugs: health and society in Britain since the 1960s. Basingstoke, UK: Palgrave Macmillan.

Moskalewicz, J., & Welbel, M. (2013). Walking through mud; history of the Polish methadone maintenance treatment from its stakeholders' perspective. *Substance Use & Misuse*, **48**, 977–996.

Orts, E.W., & Strudler, A. (2002). The ethical and environmental limits of stakeholder theory. *Business Ethics Quarterly*, **12**(2), 215–233.

Rivera, L. (2003). Changing women: an ethnographic study of homeless mothers and popular education. *Journal of Sociology and Social Welfare*, **30**(2), 31–51.

Sabatier, P., & Jenkins-Smith, H. (1993). Policy change and learning. Boulder, CO: Westview.

Sabatier, P., & Jenkins-Smith, H. (1999). The advocacy coalition framework: an assessment. In P. Sabatier (Ed.), Theories of the policy process. Boulder, CO: Westview. 117–168.

Socialministeriet. (1998). Vejledning om: Den sociale indsats for de mest udsatte voksne. Sindslidende, stof og alkoholmisbrugere, hjemløse m. fl. Lov om social service: Socialministeriet.

Stone, D. (2012). Agents of knowledge. In L. Faur (Ed.), The Oxford handbook of governance. Oxford: Oxford University Press. 339–352

Thom, B., Duke, K., Frank, V.A., & Bjerge, B. (2013). Stakeholders in opioid substitution drug user treatment policy: similarities and differences in six European countries. *Substance Use & Misuse* (48), 933–942.

Thom, B., Herring, R., Thickett, A., & Duke, K. (2015). The Alcohol Health Alliance: the emergence of an advocacy coalition to stimulate policy change. Manuscript submitted for publication.

Tops, D. (2006). Stretching the limits of drug policies: an uneasy balancing act. In J. Anker et al. (Eds.), Drug users and spaces for legitimate action. Helsinki: NAD (Nordic Council for Alcohol and Drug Research). 61–83.

Torfing, J. (1999). Workfare with welfare: recent reforms of the Danish welfare state. *Journal of European Social Policy*, **9**(5), 5–28.

Valenta, M., & Berg, B. (2010). User involvement and empowerment among asylum seekers in Norwegian reception centres. *European Journal of Social Work*, **13**(4), 483–501.

Van Hout, M.C., & McElrath, K. (2012). Service user involvement in drug treatment programmes: Barriers to implementation and potential benefits for client recovery. *Drugs: Education, Prevention and Policy*, **19**(6), 474–483.

Villadsen, K. (2008). Freedom as self-transgression: transformations in the 'governmentality' of social work. *European Journal of Social Work*, **11**(2), 93–104.

Vohnsen, N.H. (2011). Absurdity and the sensible decision [doctoral dissertation]. Aarhus: Aarhus University.

Zibbell, J.E. (2004). Can the lunatics actually take over the asylum? reconfiguring subjectivity and neo-liberal governance in contemporary British drug treatment policy. *International Journal of Drug Policy*, **15**, 56–65.

Zobel, F. (2014). Drug policy profile: AUSTRIA. European Monitoring Centre for Drugs and Drug Addiction. EMCDDA Papers, Publication Office of the European Union, Luxembourg.

Chapter 7

External influences on national drug policies in four European countries at the turn of the twenty-first century

Franca Beccaria, Jacek Moskalewicz, Vibeke Asmussen Frank, Irmgard Eisenbach-Stangl, and Sara Rolando

7.1 External influences and drug policies

In this chapter we study external influences on national drug policies in four European countries. The concept of 'external influences' refers to all influences coming from outside a national system which affect official policy and governance related to drug use. External influences may be divided into external *frameworks* such as EU directives, strategies, WHO policy programmes, and UN conventions, on the one hand, and external *stakeholders* such as foreign governments, international agencies, and NGOs, on the other.

National drug policies are particularly sensitive to external frameworks as they must operate within the scope imposed by the United Nations (UN) conventions. The implementation of these conventions is carefully monitored by UN agencies, but also by individual countries such as the United States, which not only contributes the lion's share to the UN budget, but has its own global drug policy interests. While all countries that are signatories to UN conventions have to introduce their principles, there is still some room for developing different kinds of drug policies in individual countries (e.g. in relation to severity of sanctions and different rules for possession and consumption). In addition to the UN agencies and individual countries, there are a number of other global or continental stakeholders that can play the role of external stakeholders in different countries and historical periods, such as European Monitoring Centre on Drugs and Drug Addiction (EMCDDA), Open Society Foundation, Global Drug Policy Commission (GDPC), and Harm Reduction International (HRI).

Some of these organizations, such as the HRI and the GDPC, have represented strong voices in the drug debate; others, like the EMCDDA, have held the status of epistemic communities that channel and uphold knowledge and beliefs that underpin drug policy. Epistemic communities are networks of professionals (such as members of international scientific societies) with recognized expertise and authoritative claims to policy-relevant knowledge and who typically share a set of normative and causal beliefs, so that they can influence the coordination of state policies (Haas, 1992, p. 3). In order 'to pass or to maintain a law, policymakers need to win sufficient support of it within their constituency and among stakeholders' (Alasuutari & Qadir, 2014, p. 72). Such support is sought through processes that are referred to as *epistemic work*. These involve discursive techniques used by actors engaged in 'affecting views and hegemonic definitions of the situation at hand' (ibid.). Often, the authority and experience of other countries are imitated in order to win a hegemonic position in national discourse.

In this chapter we look at how external influences, in terms of both external frameworks and stakeholders, affect national policies, and in particular how they are referred to in epistemic work to construct what the world around drugs is all about, and what is proper, evidence-based, and desirable policy and practice in this area. (For an in-depth treatment of stakeholder theory, see Chapter 5 by Houborg et al., in this volume.)

7.2 Three theoretical frameworks

Our approach intends to contribute to theories on the development of drug policies by explaining the different roles that external frameworks or stakeholders can play at the national level, offering examples from several European countries. Through reporting a number of national cases, we will expose some relationships between external influences, on the one hand, and national policies and bodies, on the other.

In order to better understand the role of external influences in the governance of drug problems, we combine three theoretical frameworks: Kingdon's 'policy windows' theory (1984), Gieryn's boundary work theory (1983), and Wiener's 'social arena' perspective (1981).

According to Kingdon's theory of agenda setting, the development of policy is the outcome of three sets of processes or 'streams': the 'problem stream', the 'policy stream', and the 'political stream'. The problem stream refers to those issues that become recognized and defined as important or significant problems that require attention by policy makers. The policy stream refers to the dominating frameworks of governance or models of change developed by policy actors based on their power and interest in particular issues. The political stream relates to the wider political environment and includes elections, swings in public opinion, ministerial changes, and interest group lobbying (Kingdon, 1984). At critical junctures, the three streams merge and 'policy windows' open; shifts or transitions in policy can occur. When policy windows open, policy entrepreneurs can seize the opportunity to push alternative ideas and policy frameworks to tackle particular problems. In this context, external influences may play a role in persuading key stakeholders to recognize problems and view them in terms of their perspective or ideological position (Kingdon, 1995). Therefore national stakeholders may look for support from external frameworks and stakeholders in order to bring the problem or issue onto the agenda within a framework which serves their particular interests. Applying Kingdon's windows theory permits us to identify the conditions under which national stakeholders can successfully place and negotiate a space for their ideas on the agenda under the influence of external forces.

Furthermore, external stakeholders—especially those represented by scientists and epistemic communities—provide alternative repertoires to be exploited for public description of a problem, as 'interests guide the selection of one or another repertoire for public presentation' (Gieryn, 1983, p. 792) depending on the circumstance. According to Gieryn's boundary-work theory, demarcation between science and non-science is not only an analytical matter, but also (or mainly) a matter of interest for scientists considered as stakeholders, as 'ideological efforts by scientists to distinguish their work from non-scientific intellectual activities' (Gieryn, 1983, p. 782). This demarcation always implies material opportunities and professional advantages so that scientists construct appropriate ideologies to gain benefits or protection of their professional authority. In this perspective ideologies are regarded as affected both by interests and strains, which guide the selection of alternative repertoires to be used for the public presentation of science on the basis of different circumstances. Boundary-work can act through the *expansion* of authority or expertise into domains claimed by other professions; *monopolization*, by excluding rivals labelled as outsiders such as 'pseudo', 'deviant', or 'amateur'; and finally the *protection of autonomy* over professional activities, relieving members from responsibility of consequences of their work by 'putting the blame on scapegoats from outside' (Gieryn, 1983, pp. 791–792).

It is not only the extent of the harms that explains why some problems get recognition and attention by policymakers and enter into the political discourse (Hilgartner & Bosk, 1988). In order to understand the process of social construction of the problem, Wiener (1981) identifies three components that lead to a collective definition of a social problem. *Animating the problem* consists of creating a ground for the problem by establishing a turf of rights, developing constituencies, funnelling advice, and imparting skills and information in order to enable further steps of *legitimizing* and *demonstrating the problem. Legitimizing the problem* occurs by 'borrowing prestige and expertise from other arenas', 'lessening the attached stigma', 'building respectability in the eyes of those outside the arena', and creating, for example, an autonomous arena for alcohol problems separated from other drug and mental health problems. *Demonstrating the problem* is a process that requires competing for attention, selecting supportive data, enlarging the bounds of respectability, and convincing opposing ideologists (Wiener, 1981, p. 73).

Through these theoretical lenses, we will examine national cases from Austria, Denmark, Italy, and Poland that include illustrative accounts of external influences and show how external frameworks and stakeholders in specific time periods interacted with national drug policies and influenced the decision-making processes. These are not complete analyses of all external influences that a country has been under, but examples of how to research and analyze them. After analyzing specific cases from these four countries, we will discuss what were the main external frameworks and stakeholders and how they played a role in shaping drug policies in certain historical periods. Finally we will suggest some implications and ideas for future research.

Each national case represents a different part of Europe with unique political, economic, and social contexts. Austria, which is geographically situated between Western and Eastern Europe, has shrunk in the last century from an empire covering almost 700,000 square kilometres to a relatively small country with a strong national identity but with clear traces of a multicultural past. Being a neutral country in military terms, Austria joined the EU relatively late, in 1995, and preserves its welfare state policy despite the neoliberal economic context that has dominated in Europe in the last two decades.

Denmark belongs to a group of Nordic countries where the welfare model is very much combined with economic equality. The Danish Gini index, which measures the level of economic inequality, is the lowest in the EU. Denmark was among the founding members of NATO and joined the EU in 1972.

Italy is a founding member of both NATO and the EU. Since the end of the World War II, it has undergone substantial economic development, which led to the establishment of the Italian welfare state. This specific welfare state is defined as 'particularistic' because it is based on the status of the worker and on a paternalistic culture, most of the time under the rule of the Christian Democrats but also under a strong presence of socialist and communist parties. Despite the recent political governmental changes that left behind the Berlusconi quasi-technocratic government, Italy remains in an unstable political situation combined with economic insecurity, including high levels of debt and growing unemployment rates.

Poland, after more than four decades of autocratic rule and a centrally planned economy, underwent a quick transition to a multiparty system and market economy. After a few years of dramatic economic recession, Poland has been on the path of economic growth. A number of problems related to the previous regime and economy of shortage (Kornai, 1982) dissolved, but new problems emerged, such as growing economic and social inequalities, social exclusion, unemployment, and poverty. Poland joined NATO in 1999 and the EU in 2004.

All in all, our sample includes representation from the Nordic countries, Mediterranean countries, as well as two central European countries which for half a century were located on opposite sides of the Iron Curtain. Against this brief general backdrop, the next sections will discuss particular aspects of the drug policies in the individual countries. We will focus on examples within recent decades but with some important excursions into the history which help to foster understanding of contemporary developments.

7.3 External influences in four countries' drug policies

7.3.1 Austria: national drug policies defended against external influences

External influences in Austrian drug policy have a long history. As part of the peace treaty after World War I, which was lost by the Austrian-Hungarian empire, Austria was forced to sign the international opium conventions and to issue regulations on narcotic substances. Within three years after World War II, when the country was occupied by the Allies and economically dependent on the United States, Austria signed the latest international drug conventions and amended its domestic regulations. Without any parliamentary discussion, further substances and possession of drugs for individual use came under control, and sentences were increased dramatically. In both cases, the U.S.—the leading stakeholder and proponent of strict drug controls—seemed to have played the main prompter role. In both cases, Austrian decision makers were in a powerless position and the changes in the national drug policy documents were substantial. Nevertheless, although the changes were dramatic, they had hardly any practical consequences: since Austria did not have significant drug problems at the time, the new regulations were rarely applied. When drug consumption and related problems increased—especially at the end of the 1960s—drug policy and legislation were quickly modified in line with traditional national concepts of replacing penalties by medical control and treatment.

The drug policy profile of Austria, recently published by the EMCDDA (Zobel, 2014), mentions that one of the leading principles of measures taken against consequences of illicit substances consumption is 'treatment instead of punishment'. Alternative responses to penal sanctions were introduced in 1971 when the 'international drug wave' arrived in the country where drug use was the habit of well-educated youth. Diversions from penal sanctions were broadened during the following decades and applied to an increasing percentage of drug offenders. The percentage of unconditional convicted drug offenders among all registered dropped continually since the 1970s; in 2014, it was 7 per cent, and about half of these sentences were fines (Report on the Drug Situation, 2014).

Substitution treatment was officially acknowledged in 1987. As with other drug-related measures, it is based on the understanding of drug consumption and related problems as a (chronic) disease. The number of drug users given substitution treatment increased quickly, and by the 1990s substitution was the treatment of choice—outside as well as in prison. Due to a constantly lowered threshold, to growing generosity in dispensing, and to an increasing involvement of GPs, the substitution programme covered one-third of problem drug users at the turn of the millennium. But the attraction of the programme to drug users as well as to drug professionals also has to be examined in the context of the substance mostly prescribed—slow-release morphine, effective for twenty-four hours, produced by a foreign company specializing in the production of opioid-containing medicines, whose Austrian branch is responsible for the retail of its products in Central Eastern Europe.

The substitution regulations enforced since 1987 protected the freedom of medical doctors to choose the drugs prescribed, similar to the treatment of other diseases, and only exceptionally recommended certain selected substances. When slow-release morphine became available in 1998 and acknowledged as a substitution substance (not only in Austria, but in other countries such as Bulgaria, Slovenia, and Spain), practitioners favoured the previously mentioned product of the foreign company, which already at the turn of the millennium took the lead on the list of substitution drugs in the country. But the slow-release morphine, as well as other substitution drugs in other countries, started to be sold on the illicit market and increasingly replaced heroin on the drug menu of users (Eisenbach-Stangl et al., 2008).

The prominent position of slow-release morphine on the illicit drug market prompted the intervention of the International Narcotics Control Board (INCB) of the UN, based in the Vienna International Centre since 1980. The Vienna International Centre is an important contributor to the national economy, and its political importance should also be recognized: its founder, Bruno

Kreisky, followed a policy of active neutrality during the Cold War and considered the centre a component and symbol of national security. The INCB noted in its annual report of 2004 'that there have been reports in Austria of the diversion of slow-release oral morphine . . . [to the illicit drug market]'. It demanded 'respective investigations' and expressed appreciation of 'being informed promptly of the results of that investigation and if necessary, of action taken by the authorities to prevent such diversion' (United Nations, 2005, p. 16). International attention was preceded by a fierce debate on the issue at the national level, mostly carried out among substitution doctors. Critics of slow-release morphine were blamed for provoking international intervention employing powerful external allies.

The Austrian government—at that time in the international floodlight due to the activities of the right-wing party—calmed the international and national debates by the immediate establishment of a working group on substitution treatment, and by a (closed) hearing in 2005, to which the foreign pharmaceutical company—the producer of the slow-release morphine—was 'invited' and partly treated as the accused. Moreover, an amendment to the substitution regulations was passed in 2006. The amendment listed substitution drugs of 'first choice', not including the slow-release morphine, but allowed ('when incompatible') the prescription of 'other drugs'. It also tightened the dispensing regulations and introduced training obligations for substitution doctors. Simultaneously, the responsibilities of the producer for monitoring side effects of the use of the substitution substance were raised.

Despite the international and national furore raised by the controversy, no significant changes in practice were observed. Moreover, the decree of 2006, which was mostly a change on paper, was amended two years later, mitigating some of the aggravation it had brought about. The prescribing and marketing of slow-release morphine remained about the same. The international and national collisions thus resulted in stricter controls but did not stop or even interrupt the process of medicalization of drug-related problems and the normalization of treatment initiated decades earlier.

Thus, in both recent and earlier decades, the 'Austrian way' was successfully defended against external influences. In all episodes, it was more or less explicitly understood and presented as the more responsive one in regard to users' needs as well as to the nature of the problem, and opposed to the 'international' approach based on deterrence. Insofar as the political responses which were opposed touched the question of 'what works effectively?', the boundary created was also one between science and beliefs or prejudices (Gieryn, 1983).

The theoretical framework sheds light on another aspect of the Austrian case: the changing position of the external influences, their definitional power, and the changing nature of the national (definition) defence. After the world wars, Austria was powerless—external definitions had not been legitimized or demonstrated, but just enforced and reinforced (components that should be added to Wiener's theory); they would only be replaced by internal definitions decades later. With the right-wing party in parliament, Austria was in an exposed position at the turn of the millennium, but as a member of EU and host of the UN office, it was also part of the external influence that got involved in the national definition process by national stakeholders.

7.3.2 **Denmark: 'resistance' against subordination**

The UN bodies and conventions have played important roles in developing Danish drug policy. Despite a lively discussion in the late 1990s, treatment initiatives were rejected by the Ministry of Health as not politically acceptable, with a reference to the INCB and to UN conventions. In particular, it was argued that heroin is not to be used in treatment for addiction (Houborg, 2010) and that safe injection sites would violate the Danish obligations as a signatory to the UN conventions (Houborg & Frank, 2014). Houborg (2010) and Houborg and Frank (2014) have shown how bureaucrats in the Ministry of Health used INCB and UN convention policies to resist implementation of heroin-assisted treatment and safe injection sites. The INCB has thus played a major role in Denmark by not allowing safe injection sites until 2012 (Houborg & Frank, 2014, p. 4).

Nevertheless, Denmark is a country with a history of more liberal—by international standards—drug policy, which lasted until 2004. The liberal policy was characterized by a depenalization of possession of cannabis for personal use from 1969 to 2003, and hence a division between 'hard' and 'soft' drugs, and a deliberate distinction between drug dealers and drug users. However, a change to a more restrictive drug policy was framed and inspired by U.S. policy. The rhetoric of the 2003 Danish policy brief 'fight against drugs' was taken from the U.S. 'war on drugs'. The thirty-five years of depenalization were revoked. Laws became more restrictive and penalties were raised for drug offences. In particular, the situation in Danish prisons was tightened: sanctions were introduced not only against possession of illegal drugs, but also their consumption (sanctions included withdrawal of leave and no possibility for early release; Frank & Kolind, 2008). That change, which reintroduced penalties for possession of drugs for personal use, is interesting since other EU countries (e.g. Portugal) at that time were moving towards decriminalization and depenalization. This illustrates how it is possible for governments to create very different policies with reference to different concurrent streams in the international sphere.

Despite external pressures for restrictive measures, the harm reduction movement has influenced the development of Danish treatment and social care systems implemented to help drug users. Since the late 1980s, and especially the late 1990s, harm reduction initiatives such as needle and syringe exchange, street-level nursing, drop-in centres, hostels for the homeless, low-threshold methadone treatment (Asmussen & Dahl, 2002)—and, since 2010 and 2012, heroin-assisted treatment and safe injection sites, respectively—have been implemented in many larger cities in Denmark (Houborg, 2012; Houborg & Frank, 2014; Houborg et al., 2014). It is difficult to say whether any organization such as Harm Reduction International (HRI) has directly influenced Danish policy. Nevertheless, stakeholders in the drug treatment field (e.g. doctors, psychologists, and social workers) did attend the HRI conferences, especially during the 2000s. Growing international recognition of harm reduction measures, especially in the wealthy EU countries, was well received in Danish political and social work spheres (contrary to Sweden).

Since 2004, Danish drug policy has been more dichotomized between control and treatment, with harm reduction being placed in the background (Houborg, 2010). Drug treatment policy and the whole quality assurance and monitoring systems were elaborated with inspiration from work done in the U.S. and the UK, particularly research work. In this context, the importance of European Addiction Severity Index (EuropASI) tool cannot be overestimated. International standards on substitution treatment inspired stakeholders in Denmark to 'medicalize' substitution treatment through quality assurance and evidence-based treatment. In particular, the DanRIS (Danish registration and information system) developed by Mads Uffe Pedersen at the Centre for Alcohol and Drug Research (CRF) has been very important in these trends towards quality assurance and evidence-based treatment policy. It was developed in the late 1990s and beginning of the 2000s.

Currently, the law requires that all drug treatment institutions, both private and public, have to report and offer file information on their patients/clients in DanRIS. If not, they will not have patients referred to them. A report from DanRIS is published annually, including an assessment of the severity of the clients/patients based on ASI scores. Internationally well-known treatment methods have thus been imported to Denmark, especially 'evidence-based methods' such as cognitive behavioural therapy, systemic therapy, motivational interviewing, etc. Vice versa, Denmark is becoming more of an external stakeholder for other countries; for example, in relation to heroin-assisted treatment and safe injection sites, and the experiences and results stemming from these initiatives. The peculiarity of Danish case is that the process that Wiener (1981) called 'legitimizing the problem' by borrowing experiences (in this case also the rhetoric) from other countries worked in two opposing directions: one supporting a more repressive drug regulation programme, the other more liberal policies of harm reduction and evidence-based treatment.

7.3.3 Italy: political demand for supportive American science

As in other countries, drug issues in Italy have always been a sensitive topic not only at the national level, but also for their international implications. After World War II, the international community played a major role in directing the Italian government's policies on drugs. The first laws, enacted during 1950–1951, regulated 'non-classical' drugs (i.e. barbiturates and other pharmaceutical drugs) and were a consequence of the 1948 Paris Protocol. Even more interesting is the influence of the UN in the promulgation of the first Italian Consolidation Act about drugs (Law 1041/1954). Indeed, the law had been put forward during the 1950 and 1953 UN Narcotic Drugs Committee meetings by French and Canadian representatives who complained about the Italian slowness in the prosecution and trials of drug traffickers. In the post-war period, Italy had always promptly subscribed to the international drug conventions, and took the leadership of the UN Office on Drugs and Crime (UNODC) from its foundation in 1997 until 2010.

Despite its involvement in the UN restrictive initiatives, Italy adopted relatively liberal legislation (Law 685/1975) in 1975 that did not punish the possession of small quantities of drugs for personal use. However, later on a big debate about substitution treatment arose, and the approach became more punitive and prohibitive, culminating in 1990 in the Drug Consolidation Act (Law 309/1990) that changed the way the Italian government responded to drug problems. Now both problematic users and occasional users were criminalized (Arnao, 1990). The introduction of this law had significantly negative results: the number of drug addicts and drug-related deaths increased considerably (Renda, 1999). In 1993, a national referendum rejected this repressive approach, establishing that personal consumption was an administrative violation only.

Under the Berlusconi governments, Italian drug policy returned to a more punitive approach—considering 'soft' and 'hard' drugs on the same level—and drug possession was again considered a criminal offence, with the exception of small quantities for personal use (Law 49/2006; Beccaria & Rolando, 2013). As a consequence of this punitive shift, there were significant increases in the rates of imprisonment for drug crimes and of the imprisonment of drug users (Zuffa, 2011). Furthermore, the number of heroin addicted considerably decreased in the first decade of the twenty-first century. This is an example of what Wiener (1981) defined as the selective use of data and scientific literature to demonstrate the relevance of the drug problem—especially cannabis use—and to animate the problem by imparting skills and information.

In this same period, the Italian approach to drug problems became closer to U.S. drug policies than to EU ones, appears clear by examining the organization of the national Department for Anti-drug Policies (DPA)—established during the second Berlusconi government (2001–2005)—and its scientific production.

According to the decree of the president of the Council of Ministers, the DPA has the responsibility to ensure coordination among different ministries and to support and promote the action of the government in anti-drug policies, and to function as a link between different levels of authorities—central, regional, and local—through the mechanism of the State-Regions Committee. Its responsibilities also include policy activities at the European and international levels, and disseminating scientific knowledge about different aspects of drug addiction and consumption.

The department comprises three sections: the observatory on drugs and addiction, the board (*consulta*), and the Scientific Committee. The board includes representatives of organizations working in the addictions field (public and private services, NGOs, and other relevant organizations), representatives of the central administration (DPA, ministries of the Interior, Justice, Education, and Health), and of regional governments. It is a consultation and concerted action body on anti-drug strategies and interventions. However, despite the ambitious tasks given to the board by the law, it has met only twice (both in the first year of its designation) since 2009.

The composition of the Scientific Committee provides an example of how epistemic communities can be exploited to affirm a particular public description of a problem and, consequently, to select specific solutions (Gieryn, 1983). Until 2014, the Scientific Committee had eleven members, most of them coming from abroad: six from the U.S. (including Nora Volkow, director of the National Institute on Drug Abuse [NIDA]), and one from the UK. Only one member came from an Italian university.

The eleven members of the committee included three psychiatrists, three pharmacologists/toxicologists, two neuroscientists, one neurologist, one psychologist, and one expert in internal medicine—who was the chair of the committee and the head of DPA. There was a complete lack of epidemiological, sociological, or anthropological experts, with the exception of the psychologist, who worked on neuroimaging and cognitive neuroscience.

The composition of the Scientific Committee is of particular importance as the committee is charged with steering government strategies on the basis of scientific evidence, promoting collaboration between Italian and international institutes, and providing scientific evaluation of projects submitted to the DPA for funding. If we examine the research projects funded since 2010, we can see that nine out of fifteen were on cannabis, with brain alterations and functions the main topic. Ten of the projects were on neuroscience and included the use of magnetic resonance in diagnosis and in research on brain damage. Clearly, neuroscience and imaging, especially applied to cannabis, was the main interest and concern of the DPA. Indeed, this specificity was already clear in the definition of the committee aims, which include the provision of international research and training in the 'neuroscience of addiction'. The concept of boundary work explains this process, especially the idea of 'monopolization' (Gieryn, 1983). In the composition and work of the Scientific Committee we can see monopolization of both nationality and scientific discipline, pursued by excluding Italian scientists and especially those from the social research field applying an interdisciplinary approach (Beccaria & Rolando, 2013).

7.3.4 **Poland: opposite external influences shaping the drug question**

As alcohol is the favourite drug in Poland and other psychoactive substances are alien to the culture, the perception of and social response to illicit drugs in Poland have almost always been under strong pressure from external influences. However, external stakeholders were not involved directly in the first stages of development of drug addiction as a social problem in Poland in the 1970s and 1980s. Rather, they were exploited by domestic stakeholders to legitimize what were seen to be innovative management strategies at the time, such as the introduction and proliferation of the therapeutic community model and liberal legislative approaches, including the depenalization of drug possession.

At the turn of the 1980s, in the early period of transition towards a market economy and multiparty system, external stakeholders became more active in Poland. Of serious international and domestic concern at that time was the risk of an HIV epidemic among drug injectors in Poland, similar to earlier epidemics that affected injecting drug users (IDUs) in New York, Edinburgh, and elsewhere. Numerous external stakeholders, such as the WHO, UN AIDS, and Dutch and British NGOs and governments encouraged Polish partners to initiate needle exchange programmes and the distribution of free condoms. The first needle exchange programmes were launched in Poland in late 1988, just after the first HIV infections were reported among IDUs.

That immediate response could be attributed to cooperation between Polish and foreign NGOs, which provided the first disposable needles and syringes, but also to bilateral cooperation between Polish and British health authorities. During the Polish-British medical week in 1987, British colleagues shared experiences of the rapid HIV epidemic among IDUs in Edinburgh which took place a few years earlier, and recommended needle exchange programmes as a humane and pragmatic response. Therefore Polish needle exchange programmes were funded by the Ministry of Health and regional health authorities. Numerous programmes mushroomed all over Poland. As drug possession was not penalized, a hidden population of addicts did not exist; drug users were therefore not afraid of being identified and reported to the police. In less than two years, the epidemic was under control. It reached its peak in 1990 when 900 new infections were recorded; in 1991 the number dropped to 300, and since then has not increased again (Kulka & Moskalewicz, 1998).

Of particular impact was a WHO/Euro 'programme on preventing drug abuse and concomitant HIV infections for countries of Central and Eastern Europe'. The programme was adopted at the beginning of the 1990s. It offered numerous training courses which encouraged such measures as syringe exchange programmes as well as methadone maintenance, which were non-existent in that part of Europe. The first methadone maintenance service started in Warsaw in 1992 as a research project to investigate if methadone was an appropriate substitution agent for Polish heroin, which was composed of different opiates including codeine, morphine, and heroin. As expected the programme brought about significant improvement in the health status of participants and shortly afterwards two other programmes followed in Warsaw (Baran-Furga & Chmielewska, 1994). Since then, however, methadone maintenance services have hardly developed, and now no more than 10 per cent of heroin users benefit from them.

Poor development of methadone maintenance in Poland can partially be explained by the dramatic redefinition of 'drug addiction' followed by significant changes in drug legislation, both of which can be attributed to numerous external stakeholders. First, printed media had to adapt themselves to the requirements of the competitive media market shaped to a large extent by international media giants such as Axel Springer. Unlike in previous decades, the media of the 1990s sought sensational coverage, and therefore underscored the criminal aspects of drug abuse, emphasized the brutality of drug dealers, and highlighted the enormous profits generated by the illicit drug trade (Świątkiewicz & Moskalewicz, 1994). In that way the media—to use social arena concepts (Wiener, 1981)—(re)animated the problem as criminal.

Demand for more severe legislation followed, particularly by politicians of different political orientations. This new approach was legitimized by examples of zero tolerance policies worked out in such countries as the U.S. and Sweden. Liberal legislation, which was adopted in the mid-1980s, was widely criticized as inadequate in a new democratic market-oriented society. Some critics blamed the previous regime for even facilitating drug use among young people. Foreign influence also consisted of offering Polish professionals attractive training opportunities. Of particular importance were scholarships in the U.S. where Polish health professionals could learn how to tackle the problem of individual addicts in medical terms against the background of oppressive drug policies. In parallel, Polish police received intensive training from their American counterparts. Pressures for changing liberal legislation and penalizing drug possession were reinforced by the INCB, which imposed orthodox interpretations of the Vienna Convention of 1988. Arguments of the INCB were keenly repeated in Polish public debates. Reversing the former 'communist' legislation seemed to be an important condition of 'joining the family of civilized nations', as it was often referred to by popular media and politicians.

A new law 'on counteracting drug abuse' was adopted in 1997. Its penal provisions were more severe in comparison with previous legislation; possession of drugs became a crime, 'with exception of small quantities for personal use'. In less than three years, the number of drug-specific crimes tripled to reach 10,000 in 1999. This rise was used to demonstrate the seriousness of the problem and to amend the law to penalize any possession without exceptions. In the following five years, the number of drug crimes reached a peak of 70,000 annually, with the majority being possession.

In contrast to the pre-transition period, rapid transition to a market economy witnessed more direct involvement of external stakeholders in Poland. Initially, due to the influence of external public health stakeholders, Polish drug policy continued to be innovative and pragmatic, in particular in response to the risks of HIV. At the same time, other external stakeholders with high political status and power succeeded in reanimating the problem (Wiener, 1981), stressing its criminal aspects and legitimizing introduction of new drug legislation and policies which gave priority to repressive measures at the expense of harm reduction and methadone maintenance.

7.4 Conclusions

Experiences from four European countries representing different regions, various welfare traditions, as well as different drug epidemiologies show that national drug policies are not autonomous actions taken by sovereign nations, but are strongly dependent on external influences.

As summarized in Table 7.1, an important role is played by the UN agencies, which recommend different priorities in drug policy. While the INCB and, to a lesser extent, the UNODC focus on supply reduction and recommend more restrictive solutions, WHO and UN AIDS tend to recommend more liberal

Table 7.1 Key drug policy changes, external influences, and theoretical frameworks

	Key drug policy changes	The main external influences involved	Main mechanisms of influence (policy windows, boundary work, and social arena)
Austria	Imposing international drug conventions (from the 1920s)	U.S.	Occupation of Austria by the allied forces, including the U.S., led to opening of the policy window (Kingdon)
	Controlling slow-release morphine (2000s)	INCB, UNODC	Active boundary work emerged between evidence-based arguments and beliefs (Gieryn)
Denmark	Resistance to safe injection rooms and heroin-assisted treatment (1990s until 2012)	INCB	Policy window opened when the Ministry of Health used INCB and UN conventions to resist domestic pressures for change (Kingdon)
	More restrictive supply reduction measures including penalization of drug possession (2003 and onwards)	U.S.	The U.S. 'war on drugs' used to legitimize more restrictive policies (Wiener)
	Harm reduction initiatives (since 1980s) Medicalization of drug treatment (since 2000)	HRI Foreign epistemic communities	New initiatives in harm reduction and drug treatment legitimized by borrowing experiences from other countries and epistemic communities (Wiener)
Italy	Penalization of drug possession (1954)	UN	Pressure from the UN opened policy window for penalization of drug possession (Kingdon)
	Institution of Department of Anti-drug Policies (DPA) (2000s)	U.S., NIDA	Selective use of data and scientific literature to demonstrate the problem (Wiener). Boundary work through monopolization of scientific discipline in favour of neuroscience (Gieryn).
Poland	Development of harm reduction policy (late 1980s, early 1990s)	WHO, foreign governments, foreign NGOs, including HRI	Outbreak of HIV epidemic opened policy window for change (Kingdon)
	Penalization of drug possession (1997)	Foreign media, foreign governments, INCB	Media reanimated drug problem as a criminal issue (Wiener)

approaches with stress on demand and harm reduction policies. The latter are currently promoted by HRI, whose pressure is exerted during its international congresses that bring together thousands of people from all over the world to exchange their experiences and reinforce their deep belief and commitment to harm reduction (Moskalewicz et al., 2007).

The UN drug conventions which claim to preserve universal moral order are imposed and monitored by superpowers, especially the most important guardian of the conventions—the United States. The U.S. could convince less powerful countries such as Austria to sign the conventions and demand their observance in individual countries, either directly or through the INCB. The U.S. exported its model of drug policy, which combines restrictive supply reduction measures with sophisticated treatment approaches. Additionally, the U.S. uses different strategies, including epistemic work, as in the U.S.-Italy relationships, and inviting scientists, professionals, policy makers, and politicians for study visits and offering them training and scholarships, as in the case of Poland in the 1990s.

As demonstrated through the Danish and Polish experiences, other wealthy European countries also offer their drug policy models for export purposes, often applying epistemic work to encourage colleagues from other countries to copy their advances in treatment.

External influences may aim at imposing new legal and policy agendas, reinforcing existing policies, resisting changes in current policies, or reintroducing previous policies. In this regard, experiences of the countries concerned differed. Austria has had a strategy of formal adoption of external frameworks, but then tends to return in practice to its traditional policies, which give priority to treatment over punishment. In Denmark, different domestic stakeholders employ external ones to resist revisions or to introduce changes in domestic policies, which, in recent decades, evolved from more liberal supply control towards more repressive approaches and medicalization. Italy put aside its own multidisciplinary scientific community by exploiting foreign epistemic communities, specifically from NIDA in the U.S., in order to get support for the neuroscientific explanation of drug consumption. Finally, in Poland, external pressures were keenly adopted by some domestic stakeholders to force their dominant vision of drug policy, which shifted from a focus on demand and harm reduction to a more repressive approach.

Figure 7.1 shows in a simplified way how external influences may affect national drug policies. The external influences are divided into external frameworks and external stakeholders which can exert pressures on domestic stakeholders or reduce their freedom to make policy choices. On the other hand, however, domestic stakeholders often exploit external stakeholders, using their authority and power to legitimize or to impose their own agenda (i.e. to

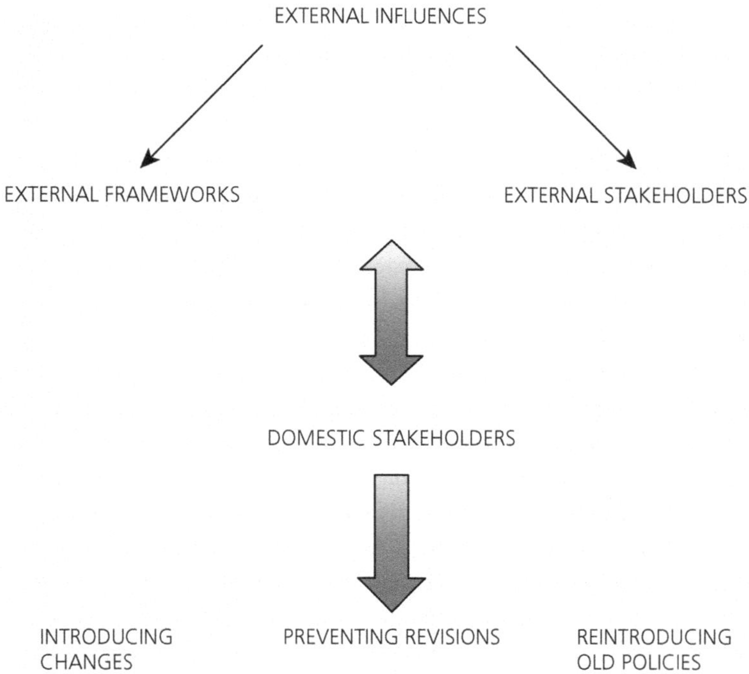

Fig. 7.1 Model of external influences.

introduce changes in drug policy, to resist revisions demanded by other domestic stakeholders, or to reintroduce old policies).

A number of theoretical perspectives need to be applied to understand better the interplay between external and domestic frameworks and stakeholders in shaping national drug policies. The major assumption of Kingdon's (1984/1995) theory—that policy windows open when political, problem, and policy streams merge around the same time—is not entirely confirmed by empirical evidence provided in this chapter. As shown by experiences from Austria, Italy, and Poland, powerful political pressure from abroad proved to be sufficient to impose UN conventions or their tough interpretation and to initiate often radical changes in drug policies at the national level. In this context, the problem stream seems to be of lesser importance, as shifts in drug policies may happen without any significant changes in drug epidemiology. Nevertheless, the problem stream may be awakened by changes in public perception of the problem, its (re)animating and demonstrating (to borrow concepts from Wiener's work on building the arena around social problems) (Wiener, 1981). In Poland, the drug problem was reanimated in the beginning of the 1990s. An image of the drug addict as an innocent victim of intergenerational conflict was redrawn by politicians and the media to show American images of addicts as criminals prepared to do anything to acquire drugs. This reanimation eventually led to the criminalization of drug possession. Imposition of a policy change by the political stream only, however, without problem and policy streams, may be short-lived. Austrian experience shows that changes may be formally adopted, as in the conflict with the INCB on slow-release morphine, but then rejected in practice where previous routines continue to be applied.

In Italy, the problem of drugs was redefined. Attempts were made to reduce it to a question of neurotransmission at the molecular level, thus shifting attention from structural determinants of social problems, which was in line with general transformations in Italian politics and their implications for health and social policies. It is important to stress the cooperation between Italy (DPA) and the U.S. (NIDA) and the role played by scientists involved in this alliance in promoting a partial, specialized view of the problem—that is, the neuroscientific approach. This can be seen as a selective use of scientific data, building up to create a social problem (Wiener, 1981). The problem was animated and demonstrated due to involvement of American scientists whose prestige was borrowed to increase the position of biomedical research and to obtain scientific legitimization of policy changes. Here Gieryn's (1983) boundary work theory can be employed to understand competition between different fields of research, in which (some) scientists use external stakeholders in order to expand their 'authority or expertise into domains claimed by other professions or occupations' (p. 791). Boundary theory also illuminates how spaces between scientific knowledge and political arguments are blurred to legitimize policy turns on the one hand, but serve the interests of some researchers or fields of science at the expense of other researchers or scientific perspectives, on the other.

The Danish experience is of particular interest, as the Danish domestic stakeholders used the authority of external influences both to resist policy change and to introduce it. External stakeholders did not impose their solutions on the problem but were carefully selected by domestic stakeholders to support their particular interests or opinions. In the late 1990s, the Health Ministry bureaucracy used the authority of UN conventions and the INCB to reject the introduction of safe injection rooms. On the other hand, tightening of drug control policies, including penalization of drug possession, was legitimized by the rhetoric of the American 'war on drugs'. Paradoxically, the authority of other countries eventually strengthened the harm reduction wing of drug policy, including the introduction of safe injection rooms and heroin-assisted treatment. Parallel to more restrictive control policies, more sophisticated and expensive treatment approaches were introduced and legitimized by advances in medical sciences in the U.S. and other countries.

The experiences of the four countries presented in this chapter indicate the theoretical usefulness of an external-influences perspective in understanding changes in national health and welfare policies. Traces of external pressures are easy to identify and track, as usually external and domestic stakeholders do not hide their positions, which often are ostensibly used to force or resist policy change. It is clear from our case studies that rarely do external stakeholders impose their policy or legal agenda directly. More frequently, domestic stakeholders employ external stakeholders or use external frameworks to introduce or resist policy change. Wiener's (1981) social arena theory exposes some strategies used by domestic stakeholders—such as animating and demonstrating the problem by borrowing foreign images of addiction, and legitimizing policy claims by advocating political solutions from other apparently more experienced countries. Gieryn's (1983) theory explains how domestic stakeholders expand their authority and monopolize scientific knowledge due to involvement of external stakeholders.

This chapter also shows that a number of theoretical approaches can be applied to explore complex issues such as drug policy changes, which are interwoven into the political, social, and moral fabrics of societies. An eclectic approach, therefore, proved to be fruitful. In addition to their pragmatic or functional dimensions, drug policies have powerful symbolic meanings. Within the national states they may reflect political and moral struggles between opposite ideological camps and important shifts in power and wealth, but sometimes drug policies may represent the expression of national consensus against external pressures. In international relationships, changes in drug policy often reflect not only political alliances but also power relationships between countries.

7.5 **Acknowledgements**

Section 7.3.1 (Austria) is based on the analysis of laws, scientific literature, and other material (e.g. statistics), partly summarized in other publications (mainly Eisenbach-Stangl, 2014), and on an interview with representatives of the pharmaceutical company mentioned in the text and on their written responses to the questions from the guidelines drafted especially for the interview. Most of reported information about the DPA in Section 7.3.3 (Italy) was retrieved from the official website (http://www.politicheantidroga.it, retrieved October 2014) and elaborated by the authors. At the time of writing, the website was being updated as the director changed. Nevertheless, it was possible to access the web archive: http://web.archive.org/web/20130609104738/ and http://www.politicheantidroga.it/organismi/comitato-scientifico.aspx.

References

Alasuutari, P., & Qadir, A. (2014). Epistemic governance: an approach to the politics of policy making. *European Journal of Cultural and Political Sociology*, **1**(1), 67–84.

Arnao, G. (1990). Proibito capire: proibizionismo e politiche di controllo sociale. Torino: Ed. Gruppo Abele.

Asmussen, V., & Dahl, H.V. (2002). Skadesreduktionsomforebyggelsepåstofmisbrugsområdet. *NordiskAlkohol-ogNarkotikatidsskrift*, **19**(4), 249–261.

Baran-Furga, H., & Chmielewska, K. (1994). Terapia metadonem. *Alkoholizm i Narkomania*,**15**(1), 25–43.

Beccaria, F., & Rolando, S. (2013). Stakeholders' role in contemporary 'substitute drug' prescribing policies in Italy. *Substance Use & Misuse*, **48**(11), 943–953.

Eisenbach-Stangl, I. (2014). Deviance or innovation? Recent changes of drug substitution treatment policy in Austria. *Substance Use & Misuse*, **48**, 1010–1021.

Eisenbach-Stangl, I., Moskalewicz, J., & Thom, B. (Eds). (2008). Two worlds of drug consumption in late modern societies. Farnham: Ashgate.

Frank, V.A., & Kolind, T. (2008). Dilemmas experienced in prison-based cannabis treatment—drug policy in Danish prisons. In V.A. Frank et al. (Eds.), Drug policy: history, theory and consequences. Aarhus: Aarhus University Press. 61–86.

Gieryn, T. (1983). Boundary-work and the demarcation of science from non-science: strains and interests in professional ideologies of scientists. *American Sociological Review*, **48**, 781–795.

Haas, P. (1992). Introduction: epistemic communities and international policy coordination. *International Organization*, **46**(1), 1–35.

Hilgartner, S., & Bosk, C.L. (1988). The rise and the fall of social problems: a public arenas model. *American Journal of Sociology*, **94**, 53–78.

Houborg, E. (2010). Control and welfare in Danish drug policy. *Journal of Drug Issues*, **40**(4), 783–804.

Houborg, E., & Frank, V.A. (2014). Drug consumption rooms and the role of politics and governance in policy processes. *International Journal of Drug Policy*, **25**(5), 972–977.

Houborg, E., Frank, V.A., & Bjerge, B. (2014). From zero tolerance to non-enforcement: creating a new space for drug policing in Copenhagen, Denmark. *Contemporary Drug Problems*, **41**(2), 261–291.

Houborg, E. (2012). The political pharmacology of methadone and heroin in Danish drug policy. *Contemporary Drug Problems*, **39**(1), 155–192.

Kingdon, J. (1995). Agendas, alternatives and public policies (2nd ed.). Boston: Little Brown. (1st ed. 1984)

Kornai, J. (1982). Growth, shortage, and efficiency: a macrodynamic model of the socialist economy. Berkeley: University of California Press.

Kulka, Z., & Moskalewicz, J. (1998). Wpływ wymiany igieł i strzykawek na zakażenia HIV wśród narkomanów opiatowych w Polsce. *AlkoholizmiNarkomania*, **30**(1), 29–40.

Moskalewicz, J., Barret, D., Bujalski, M., Dąbrowska, K., Klingemann, H., Klingemann, J., Malczewski, A., & Struzik, M. (2007). Harm reduction coming of age: a summary of the '18th International Conference of the Reduction of Drug Related Harm' Warsaw, Poland, 13–17 May 2007. *International Journal of Drug Policy*, **18**(6), 503–508.

Renda, E. (1999). Droga: immaginario e realtà. Roma: Armando.

Report on the Drug Situation 2014 (2014). Vienna: Österreichisches Bundesinstitut für Gesundheitswesen.

Świątkiewicz, G., & Moskalewicz, J. (1994). Changing definitions of the drug problems; an analysis of Polish news-papers in 1985 and 1990–1993 period. In M. Lagerspetz (Ed.), Social problems in newspapers: studies around the Baltic Sea. Helsinki: Nordic Council for Alcohol and Drug Research. 71–82.

United Nations. (2005). Report of the International Narcotics Control Board for 2004. Washington: United Nations Publications.

Wiener, C. (1981). The politics of alcoholism: building an arena around a social problem. New Brunswick, NJ: Transaction Books.

Zobel, F. (2014). Drug policy profile: AUSTRIA, European Monitoring Centre for Drugs and Drug Addiction, EMCDDA Papers, Publication Office of the European Union.

Zuffa, G. (2011). How to determine personal use in drug legislation: the 'threshold controversy' in the light of Italian experience. *Legislative Reform of Drug Policies*, **15**, 1–11. Retrieved 4 November 2014. http://www.druglawreform.info/en/publications/legislative-reform-series-/item/2710-how-to-determine-personal-use-in-drug-legislation

Chapter 8

Underpinnings of tobacco policy: an epistemic governance perspective

Matilda Hellman, Pekka Hakkarainen, and Gunnar Sæbø

8.1 Tobacco control as a case study

The first episode of the hit American TV series *Mad Men* is set in the year 1960. In it, the advertising agency Sterling Cooper gets a visit from representatives of the makers of the cigarette brand Lucky Strike. They want to launch a new advertising campaign to counter the effects of a report saying that smoking can lead to various health issues, including lung cancer (Baglia & Foster, 2014; Wikipedia, 2014).

This is absolutely a credible scenario: in real life, the 1960s was the decade when new evidence of the relationship between tobacco smoking and health hazards started to reach the attention of the public in the USA and Europe. In 1961, the American Cancer Society, the American Heart Association, the National Tuberculosis Association, and the American Public Health Association sent a joint letter to President Kennedy, pointing out the increasing evidence of the health hazards of smoking and urging the president to establish a commission. In 1962, a report from the British Royal College of Physicians was the first to document a causal relationship between smoking and cancer (Royal College of Physicians, 1962). Despite the mounting evidence of smoking's adverse effect on health and life expectancy, it remained a common pastime in all urbanized environments in Western societies for at least twenty-five years.

The authors of this chapter assume that Norwegian and Finnish advertising agents may have smoked indoors throughout the 1960s, 1970s, and 1980s to the same extent as their fictive American colleagues in the *Mad Men* series. However, by the mid-1990s, Norway and Finland, like many other Western countries, had adopted laws to limit smoking to spatially restricted areas. Work places, restaurants, trains, and other public spaces were to be smoke-free.

Smoking was allowed only in specially designated areas and rooms. Twenty years later, in the late 2010s, tobacco smoking is prohibited in just about every indoor space, and is a rather rare sight in the streets of Helsinki and Oslo.

The different concerns raised by the fictive tobacco brand representatives along with American and British public health bodies mark the beginning of an era of tobacco control which came to entail and reflect great social change. Tobacco policies have helped create the current strong imperative for tobacco-free spaces. By denormalizing smoking behaviour, tobacco control has also fitted into, and reflected, wider societal processes, such as medicalization and individualization and changes in associated health values (Chapman & Freeman, 2008). These changes have been coordinated on a global scale through knowledge production and circulation, through opinion formation by scientific and other institutions, by cultural mediators, and by the media.

The tobacco question can be seen as a rather clear-cut case of global governance of so-called epistemic power, which works by making actors perceive the world similarly on the basis of evidence and adherent argument constructs (Alasuutari & Qadir, 2014; IPSA, 2014). By epistemic governance, we mean a set of interrelated processes that describe how actors act upon each other's conceptions, aspirations and motivations, how mentalities and government in a Foucauldian sense are fused. Epistemic work works through three objects: (a) ontology of the environment (notions about truth, facts, what is); (b) actors and identifications (self-understandings, identities, rituals), and (c) norms and ideals (notions about rights and duties). Alasuutari and Qadir (2014) have argued that the study of these aspects of epistemic work in public policies will inevitably unmask how society is governed through actors' perceptions of the world.

Epistemic governance thus refers to an evidence-based, yet tacit, homogenizing of polices across socio-geographical space. The forces that drive such convergence in understandings include nation states, domestic stakeholders, the media, regional organizations, IGOs, and INGOs (IPSA, 2014; see also neoinstitutional work such as Beck et al., 2012; Koo & Ramirez, 2009; Meyer, 2008). In this chapter we describe some stages of tobacco control and related developments in epistemic governance in our own countries, Norway and Finland. We are especially interested in the ways in which values of health and welfare are upheld by evidence of influential epistemic communities (transnational networks of knowledge experts in public health) and how this is reflected in tobacco control. Although we have chosen Norway and Finland as cases, our accounts resemble developments in other countries. Tobacco policies have followed converging lines of evidence (Proctor, 2012) in relatively similar stages in all prosperous welfare states over the last twenty-five years.

8.2 Three stages of epistemic governance

As early as the 1930s, German scientists had revealed a connection between smoking and lung cancer; smoking was strongly discouraged by a heavy government-sponsored anti-smoking campaign. These German results were rediscovered, verified, and amplified by UK and American scholars: in 1950 alone, five separate epidemiological studies were published (Proctor, 2012), including papers by Ernst Wynder and Evarts Graham (1950) in the USA and Richard Doll and A. Bradford Hill (1950) in England. All confirmed that smokers of cigarettes were far more likely to contract lung cancer than non-smokers. During the 1950s and 1960s, physicians in both Great Britain and the U.S. were warning governments of the dangers of smoking. The growing evidence base of the harms of tobacco smoking has clearly driven and justified policies, control, and governance of smoking and smokers.

Nonetheless, the arguments have had different emphases at different times. For instance, in Norway and Finland, certain ontological and epistemological traits have been tied to the increase in tobacco control since the countries' first tobacco laws were adopted in the mid-1970s. By *ontology* we mean the views on the world and reality that have permeated tobacco policy; by *epistemology* we mean the knowledge and beliefs that have permeated the same. We argue that the political developments in these countries have basically followed three steps of knowledge production concerning the danger of tobacco for the user, the harm caused to others, and the addictiveness of tobacco products (Hakkarainen, 2013). These are traits that are actively articulated by advocates pushing to mainstream epistemic governance; they have been backed up in general attitudes and 'truths' and upheld in myth and by culture. Simultaneously, agents with the power to influence historical and popular images and perceptions as well as the tobacco industry have created and marketed other images of smoking—as a cool, charming, sexy activity (Klein, 1993).

Changes in tobacco control methods have involved a certain ethics and morals (Chapman, 2007). The normatively correct ways of proceeding in tobacco control have been synchronized with an 'evidence-based moral perception' in historical contexts and settings. We will use the concept of epistemic governance (Alasuutari & Qadir, 2014) in order to discern the epistemic assumptions and logics that permeate political action in the tobacco question.

Tobacco control serves as an almost perfect case study of epistemic governance: policymaking and legislative changes have been based on scientific knowledge and it has been relatively easy to translate arguments against smoking into advocacy and concrete policy measures globally, unlike, for example, food and drink policy. The tobacco industry fought successfully for decades to counter the science on tobacco's harmful effects. The scientific community itself, they argued, was divided regarding the evidence of cause and effect, especially with respect to the relationship between smoking and cancer. Nevertheless, when the epidemiological evidence could no longer be denied, the message of the scientific community was accepted and the problem addressed more or less concurrently in all Western societies. The forces that advocated population-wide public health action to lower and control tobacco consumption and smoking have been skilful in communicating the urgency and priority of the matter. One of our arguments will be that the historical phases and nature of tobacco control have been unique. In Section 8.2.1 we discuss each stage of tobacco control's changing architecture and implementation: the basic restrictions and denormalization processes of the 1970s; raising awareness of the danger of passive smoking in the 1990s; and finally the medical and psychological assistance to people struggling to quit smoking in the era of addiction (Berridge, 1998).

8.2.1 Basic restrictions and denormalizing

The first stage of tobacco control took place at about the same time in Norway and Finland. The Norwegian *Tobacco Act* was adopted in 1975, and in Finland, the *Tobacco Act* was passed in 1976 (Tobacco Act, 1976). Like many other tobacco laws in the Western world at the time, they were the result of a documented causal influence of smoking on lung cancer and COPD in the early 1960s (Norwegian Cancer Society, 1967). At the time, smoking was culturally considered normal behaviour, a result of a free choice made by rational individuals. The aimed-for ontological stance underpinning epistemic work was to forge a consensus in government circles and public opinion on the need to reduce tobacco harm to smokers by reducing tobacco consumption (Sæbø, 2012).

The Norwegian *Tobacco Act* introduced a ban on advertising and compulsory health warnings on cigarette packets, and raised the legal age of purchase from 15 to 16. In essence, it was a harm reduction model which aimed to reduce excessive use and encourage ideas about prevention, cessation, and less harmful products that could replace tobacco. Scientifically, it acknowledged the strong positive correlation between level of consumption and risk of mortality. In Finland, the *Tobacco Act* was likewise the result of a consensus regarding the importance of restricting availability of tobacco products based on proven and obvious effects on smokers' health, but both acts also contained certain elements aimed at changing normativity of use and the cultural context of smoking. Both sought to raise the normativity threshold of consuming tobacco products and to inform consumers of the danger of smoking. The Finnish act also included a ban on tobacco advertising, compelled manufacturers to add a visible warning on tobacco packaging, limited the content of certain ingredients in tobacco, and banned the sale of tobacco to people younger than 16.

When drafting the Finnish legislation, lawmakers, according to Leppo (1978), followed four main tracks aimed at creating a health-centred tobacco policy: (a) health education, (b) price policy, (c) restrictions on availability, and (d) research and development. The committee tasked with examining the smoking problem in Norway recommended a similar approach to curbing smoking. The committee divided control measures into three types: health education; measures aimed at restricting access to tobacco; and therapeutic approaches to, for instance, smoking cessation. Although the committee had been careful when drafting the bill to emphasize the need to avoid discriminating against or provoking smokers unnecessarily, the resulting measures were chiefly restrictive and in line with a denormalization philosophy. This aim had been stated as early as 1970 in parliament, and soon became the dominant doctrine of epistemic governance of tobacco production and consumption (Sæbø, 2012).

It is interesting to note in the very basic articulation in the laws passed in the 1970s of smoking's danger to health that information and education were already at this initial stage of tobacco control viewed as matters in need of 'fixing' by denormalizing smoking socially and culturally. This denormalization process has been extensively covered in the literature on tobacco policy (Thompson et al., 2007), where there seems to be a rather widespread consensus that tobacco policy, more than other addiction policies, has rested on a discourse of repellence, with the aim of denormalizing the behaviour. According to Bell and her colleagues (2010), the denormalization strategies of tobacco control advocates have embraced the use of stigma as a policy tool and the active 'othering' of smokers.

Another interesting fact when elucidating how denormalization policies were framed in the first wave of tobacco legislation is that the literature on tobacco policy often positioned availability restrictions within the scope of the denormalization aims. Typically—for example, in alcohol policy research—the denormalization effect of availability restrictions is viewed as a secondary aim, the first being to restrict people's opportunities to ingest alcohol, argued in terms of costs and pain to society (Edwards, 1997, p. 75). Could it be that the rapid development of tobacco policies was accelerated by the denormalization philosophy that seemed to inform all sorts of initiatives?

The subject of intoxication, so important in the stigmatizing mechanisms of substance use (alcohol and narcotics), is absent in the tobacco question: there are no drunkards and junkies to thrust aside or feel sorry for. The concept of stigma that is inherently attached to those doing the stigmatizing and those being stigmatized is often restricted to the habit or the behaviour, not to the actual smoker. Could it be that the separation between the person with the habit and the actual behaviour also allowed for an early consensus on what is good and what is bad, enabling a rapid change in the drafting and adoption of restrictive measures? Addiction and dependency concepts have been particularly easy to graft onto the tobacco discourse and have allowed the idea to emerge of the distinction between the person and the habit (Benowitz, 1999; Hoffman & Slade, 1993; Stolerman & Jarvis, 1995). Partly due to the moralistic legacy from the temperance movement, alcohol consumption in Norway and Finland is always tied to the consumer (Tarnaala, 2005). It was the drinker that had to be controlled so that he wouldn't take the road home via the pub. In drug policy it is the drug taker who is inevitably the site of the drug problem (Sulkunen, 2009).

The first wave of smoking legislation and restrictions was thus based on evidence of the harm caused by smoking to the smoker, but it aimed not only to reduce smoking prevalence and smoking opportunities—it was also clearly formulated to change attitudes. Here, too, smoking policies diverge from alcohol and drug policies, something about which the epistemic community of public health experts and politicians agreed. Even the tobacco industry was at first sympathetic to the need to restrict access to tobacco products (Sæbø 2012). Although the smoker was the one affected by restrictions, it was the *habit* and the *behaviour* that were to be erased from (young) people's lives and the imagery in their environments. Still, in this initial stage, smoking was still widely accepted and viewed as normal in workplaces, bars, and restaurants.

8.2.2 **Harm to others**

In the 1990s the concept of passive smoking was added to the ontological assumptions underlying conceptions of tobacco issues. In a radically new way, it strengthened demands for tighter tobacco regulations in many countries (Jackson, 1995; Troyer, 1989). In the second big Finnish law reform, from the mid-1990s, protection against the harms of passive smoking became a central issue. New research had produced evidence of the damage caused by passive smoking to family members and co-workers (Berridge, 1999; Keane, 2002; Lesmes & Donofrio, 1992). The scope of preventive policies was therefore broadened in order to protect innocent non-smokers whose health was 'unintentionally' at risk from passive smoking. Another motivation for the reform was the widespread dissatisfaction within the public health sector regarding the lack of efficiency of some of the previous restrictive measures, such as the advertising ban. Denormalization had not worked as well as the public bodies had hoped. In Finland, smoking had not decreased as much as desired following the 1976 act (Piha, 1992; Rimpelä, 1992).

The 1990s law reform in Finland raised the minimum purchasing age to eighteen and tightened restrictions on tobacco advertising by forbidding indirect marketing. New regulations aimed at the protection of citizens against exposure to second-hand smoke included a tightening of the ban on smoking in public spaces indoors and a widening of its scope to include workplaces and environments occupied by minors under eighteen (Tobacco Act, 1994). The 1990s law reform can be seen as a move by the government to tighten its hold on three aspects of the tobacco question at a time when the science was considered incontrovertible: the danger of smoking (including addictiveness and perils for youth); the danger of passive smoking; and the importance of an official stance against smoking.

Norwegian tobacco policy too was marked by the influential 'knowledge summary' on the harmful effects of passive smoking, issued in 1986 (U.S. Department of Health and Human Services, 1986). The evidence on the harmful effects of passive smoking accelerated the introduction of further restrictive measures against smoking. Legislation on smoke-free public places (workplaces and restaurants) was first introduced in 1988, and further tightened in 1995 and 1998. The purchasing age in Norway was raised to eighteen, and indirect marketing was prohibited.

The 'harm to others' perspective thus reinforced the push to denormalize smoking. It also heralded a slight moralistic turn in legitimating further restrictions, as the distinction between smokers and non-smokers was given greater prominence and the individual's 'right to smoke' more difficult to defend. Proof of the harmful environmental effects of tobacco smoke provided much sought-after evidence for an argument the anti-tobacco campaign had been proposing since World War I (Sæbø, 2014). Eventually, a smoke-free environment became the normative ideal and prompted a vision of a totally tobacco-free environment (as later expressed by the notion of 'tobacco endgame' policies in countries like Finland and New Zealand).

These developments were also nourished by a clearer divide between health and industry interests. The tobacco industry had initially played along with the harm reduction model (analyzed in Section 8.2.1) by developing and marketing light cigarettes. These cigarettes were soon found to be just as harmful as regular cigarettes, however. And after the publication of papers revealing the manipulation and silencing of evidence by the tobacco industry in the mid-1990s (Glantz, 1996), the gap between health and industry interests evolved into an abyss. The WHO-associated 'tobacco or health' slogan united public health interests against the tobacco industry in what was aptly named a 'tobacco war' (Glantz & Balbach, 2000). Whether knowledge of tobacco's harm to others and the increasing scorn heaped onto the industry also blurred the distinction between the smoker and the behaviour remains an unanswered question, but it seems very likely.

8.2.3 The struggle to overcome nicotine dependency

The role played by medical, psychological, and social help for smokers remained rather unclear and indistinguishable in the first two major law reforms in the 1970s and 1980s (Hakkarainen, 2013; Sæbø, 2012). Indeed, it was not until the late 1980s and early 1990s, when a more specified treatment paradigm started to emerge, that nicotine addiction became a key concept in the definition of tobacco as a problem (Bell & Keane, 2012; Berridge, 1998; Elam, 2012). Here, the modern concept and idea of the phenomenon of 'addiction' played a major role. The report 'Nicotine Addiction', published by the U.S. Surgeon General in 1988, concluded that tobacco, no matter the form in which it is used, leads to addiction that is pharmacologically and behaviourally comparable to the addiction caused by hard drugs like heroin and cocaine (U.S. Department of Health and Human Services, 1988; West & Grundberg, 1991). This was a discursive event that produced the smoker as a pathological subject (Keane, 2002). In the vocabulary of epistemic governance, it created an important paradigmatic aspect that highlighted freedom and free will (good, desirable) in opposition to enslavement to a chemical substance (bad, avoidable). It is an ontological position that divides the person with the problematic habit into a benign, well-intentioned 'will' and a compulsive 'must' which inevitably will cause the person to give in to certain desires (Valverde, 1998). This fits well with our earlier suggestion that the tobacco question did not involve that many other epithets that could confuse the image of the smoker, in comparison to the intoxicated, othered, and/or marginalized substance abuser.

In Finland, the definition of nicotine addiction has widened the scope of tobacco policy by strengthening the role of treatment in tackling the tobacco problem (Hakkarainen, 2013). When the smoker is seen as a person in need of help, and not primarily a person who needs to be warned and punished, the solution to the smoking problem gains greater emphasis in support and 'treatment techniques' aimed at helping the smoker in his or her 'condition'. Indeed, the new *Tobacco Act* (2010), whose ultimate aim is a tobacco-free Finland by 2040, has three goals: to prevent people from starting to smoke, to encourage and enable smokers to quit, and to protect people from exposure to tobacco smoke. In fact, it has been stated, the stock of legal restrictions might already have been largely realized; Finnish tobacco policy should now put more emphasis on developing preventive and curative measures—areas in which Finland has been ranked below average on the European tobacco control scale (Heloma et al., 2012; Joossens & Raw, 2006).

The reconception of tobacco as an addictive drug accompanied the development of new technologies of treatment and quitting (Hakkarainen, 2013). An exciting example of a new curative method is nicotine substitution treatment (Bell & Keane, 2012; Elam, 2012). The first medical nicotine product, a chewing gum named Nicorette® (2 mg and 4 mg), was introduced into the Finnish pharmacopoeia Pharmaca Fennica in 1984. From then on, the development of these products accelerated. By 1997, nine different nicotine substitution products were marketed by big pharmaceutical companies like Pharmacia & Upjohn and Novartis in the form of chewing gum or patches (Hakkarainen, 2000). It raised the value of the nicotine product market many times over (Hakkarainen, 2000). In other words, the new conception of nicotine addiction generated a new economic interest group, the pharmaceutical industry, in the field of smoking and defining the problem. A recent trend is to prescribe antidepressants such as bupropion, varenicline, and nortriptyline as aids in smoking cessation (Tupakkariippuvuus, 2012). In health services, different short-term intervention strategies were adopted and courses on quitting were renamed curative treatment. All in all, the concept of nicotine addiction has achieved an acknowledged position in the Finnish school of medicine (Tupakkariippuvuus, 2012). '[The] dosage–response relationship holds up in treatment: the more intensive pharmacotherapy and counselling, the better the treatment outcomes', state Kinnunen and colleagues (2012, p. 3560) in a recent overview published in the *Finnish Medical Journal*.

With respect to the 'discovery' of nicotine addiction, the immediate response in Norway was to ban the import and production of new nicotine and tobacco products in 1989 (a ban that still stands). Even if the health authorities were initially a little hesitant to embrace the products of the pharmaceutical industry, the Norwegian tobacco field developed much like that of Finland in the 1990s, with greater emphasis on nicotine treatment and nicotine replacement therapy (NRT) as a cessation method. A telephone quit-line was established in 1996 (Bliksrud & Nygaard, 2002), use of NRT as a cessation method was included in official statistics from 1997 onwards, and the sale of nicotine replacement products has risen steadily and linearly since 1990 in Norway (Skretting et al., 2014, p. 152). Norway's recent national strategy against tobacco, 2013–2016, has exactly the same three policy goals as in Finland, including steps to motivate and help users quit using snuff (*snus*) and smoking (Helse- og omsorgsdepartementet [HOD], 2013, p. 12). Still, while third on the European tobacco control scale, Norway is even lower than Finland on treatment to help dependent smokers stop (Joossens & Raw, 2006).

In Finland, official attitudes to other products and measures marketed as means of reducing tobacco harm have been reserved and rather negative. As early as the 1994 tobacco law reform, Finland had banned the sale of snuff (Swedish *snus*) and took a wholesale negative attitude to tobacco products. This was consistent with the EU directive on the issue but constituted a very different stance compared to those of Finland's neighbouring countries Sweden and Norway. However, because there was almost no tradition of smokeless tobacco, the state administration in Finland—in contrast to Sweden (Örnberg, 2013)—preferred to follow the dominant European line before asking for a national exception in the EU membership negotiations (Hallituksen Esitys, 1993). The framing of Swedish *snus* as a harm reduction measure therefore never gained much hold in the epistemic governance of tobacco problem in Finland in the way that it has in Sweden and in Norway.

Another recent issue that is very much related to substitution therapy is e-cigarettes. The use of e-cigarettes is booming in many countries as it allows the habitual action of smoking without the infusion of damaging carcinogens. At the same time, experts are debating whether e-cigarettes should be categorized as tobacco products, harm reduction medication, or just consumer products providing pleasure to the user (Bell, 2013; Bell & Keane, 2012; Farsalinos & Stimson, 2014; Klein, 2013; McNeill et al., 2014). In Finland, the tobacco control movement tends to see e-cigarettes as tobacco products that are jeopardizing the strategy of a denormalization of smoking behaviour. Actually, from this point of view, e-cigarettes can be seen as a step towards the renormalization of smoking. However, following the decision of the EU Parliament, Finland is not allowed to regulate e-cigarettes through the *Tobacco Act*, only through medical legislation. While e-cigarettes are not defined as tobacco products in Finnish legislation, they are seen as replicas, and, as such, the marketing of devices and nicotine concentrates is banned by the *Tobacco Act* (Ruokolainen et al., 2014). All in all, the framing of e-cigarettes as means of reducing tobacco harm is rather rare in Finland. Consequently, the official e-cigarette policy does not support a wider use of them. In practice, devices are available in the domestic markets, but nicotine concentrates have to be ordered from abroad.

In Finland, unlike in some other countries, the development of tobacco control policy was not originally based on pressure created by wider social movements or organized, tobacco-resisting citizen groups. The initiator and driving force was the state health administration, supported by a relatively small network of tobacco control advocates (Hakkarainen, 2013). This political force followed international trends closely and applied for changes in the legislation when there were sufficient grounds and evidence to support reforms. The commonly held ideal informing the tobacco policymaking process was public health. Correspondingly, medical science and medical doctors have gained a position as leading authorities in defining the tobacco issue and tobacco problem in Finland.

The emergence and strengthening of the treatment paradigm has further reasserted the authority of the medical sphere. The general reluctance to adopt the notion of tobacco harm reduction may be related to an epistemic governance of the tobacco issue in Finland strictly based on the denormalizing strategy of smoking and nicotine addiction strongly based upon public health science.

Snus was not prohibited in Norway as it was in Finland (after Finland joined the EU), nor did Norway have to apply to the EU for an exemption to the EU ban (as Sweden had to). This is due to Norway's coupling to the inner European market via the EEA Treaty rather than via full EU membership. Given that *snus* is markedly less harmful than cigarettes, this unique situation has provided the conditions for a possible re-emergence of a harm reduction approach in Norway, though it has little support among public health officials, who have favoured a proactive approach to *snus* (even if there are individual proponents of the view within the medical field). However, the increase in *snus* use among the young has also triggered a debate on the relative risk associated with smoking and *snus*, though the official Norway is unwilling to compare the health risks of the two. The arrival of the e-cigarette may change this, however, as Norwegian health authorities have yet to decide whether to categorize and regulate e-cigarettes as pharmaceuticals, tobacco, or consumer goods (Lund, 2013). Again, Norway's association with the EU under the EEA Treaty gives Norwegian health authorities greater regulative freedom regarding e-cigarettes than the EU countries.

The concept of nicotine dependency has played a decisive role in the formation of contemporary views on tobacco use and smoking. The concept communicated initially an understanding of the dilemma between a person's intention to stop smoking and inability to succeed due to physical dependency on the nicotine. Secondarily, we can see that the idea and concept of dependency or addiction has facilitated a huge market of techniques and substitution products to aid smoking cessation. The importance of the idea of dependency in smoking control can be illustrated by the fact that 'treatment of tobacco dependency', in terms of NRT and the like, was the first item in the WHO country profiles on tobacco control (http://www.who.int/tobacco/surveillance/policy/country_profile/fin.pdf).

International authorities in the field of tobacco control have been the WHO, the U.S. surgeon general, and the Royal College of Physicians in Britain. WHO's goal-oriented messages have played a huge role (Cisneros & Sohlberg, 2012). Public health advocacy and tobacco control have, especially during the 2000s, merged into a global action paradigm permeated with the language of medicine (Chapman, 2007). In 2013, the WHO published its report on what it referred to the 'global tobacco epidemic' (the subtitle is 'Enforcing Bans on Tobacco

Advertising, Promotion and Sponsorship'). One senses the urgency to address this widespread problem in the medical language that public health officials apply to the behaviour of smoking; marketing is defined as the enabling factor in the spread of this 'bacteria'. Says the report,

> About 2.3 billion people are now covered by at least one tobacco control measure at the highest level of achievement. This is due to the actions taken by many WHO Member States to fight the tobacco epidemic. These countries can be held up as models of action for the many countries that need to do more to protect their people from the harms of tobacco use. (http://www.who.int/tobacco/global_report/2013/en/)

WHO subsequently produced an internationally applicable and now widely recognized summary of the essential elements of tobacco control strategy, published as the helpfully mnemonic MPOWER tobacco control strategy. The six components are Monitor tobacco use and prevention policies; Protect people from tobacco smoke; Offer help to quit tobacco use; Warn about the dangers of tobacco; Enforce bans on tobacco advertising, promotion, and sponsorship; Raise taxes on tobacco.

Simultaneously, the fact that NRT is not always successful among heavy smokers has raised the provocative question as to whether nicotine addiction should not perhaps be 'accepted'. Arguing that nicotine is not harmful in small doses, harm reductionists often cite Michael Russell (1976, p 1431): 'People smoke for the nicotine but they die from the tar'. As long as the nicotine is delivered via devices and technologies that are markedly less harmful than combustible tobacco—such as Swedish *snus* and e-cigarettes—why should such products not be allowed alongside NRT? If they have public health benefits, there is no reason to ban them, harm reductions argue.

The epistemic community that advises tobacco policymakers is thus divided. The ultimate objective—to which most experts, governments, and the WHO subscribe—is a smoke-free world. A minority (admittedly of influential individuals) tends to accept the idea of harm reduction. As such, the third phase we are analyzing finds the norms and ideals of the previous two phases—a smoke-free environment and harm reduction—jostling for precedence.

8.3 **Conclusions**

Today, the absence of tobacco smoking in public spaces in Norway and Finland reflects a view of smoking as a very unfortunate and dangerous habit that is strongly discouraged. While once a widespread and 'understandable' habit of the 1980s and 1990s, smoking has rapidly been removed to the fringes of socially acceptable behaviour. Historically, it is hard to find other proclivities that have been 'intentionally' manoeuvred in such a short time. The shifting

Table 8.1 The three stages of tobacco control and views of the problem

	Stage 1: 1950->	Stage 2: 1970->	Stage 3: 1990->
Ontology	Harm to self	Harm to others	Addiction
Actors	Unified	Public health vs. tobacco industry	Divide amongst PH, pharmaceutical vs. tobacco industry
Norms and ideals	Harm reduction (HR)	Smoke-free (SF)	HR vs. SF

spatial visibility of smoking over time reflects stages in legislation and tobacco policies, and levels of cultural tolerance of the habit. Table 8.1 shows the characteristics of the three stages identified in the respective tobacco policies of Finland and Norway.

The notion of causality on which the arguments in the first stage of tobacco policies were built concerned the ingestion of smoke and its harmful bodily consequences to the smoker. Total tobacco consumption gave the level of harm inflicted on the population. Normatively, smoking was attacked by restricting availability (in terms of retail outlets and purchasing age) and by limiting its commercial imagery. People were advised not to start in the first place, and smokers encouraged to stop smoking. Education and information would sensitize the public to the danger of smoking, promoting a sensibility and rationality that would steer the (potential) smoker away from the habit.

The notion of causality emphasized in the second reform stage concerned especially the health hazard of exposure to smoke by 'innocent' non-smoking third parties. A normative and moral framework was built up around the harmful influence on the passive smoker. Another important factor that was stressed was the connection between health risks and age of smoking debut. Dangerous and risky environments were identified in line with the risk discourse of the 1990s (Heloma et al., 2012). Marketing of tobacco products was seen as normalizing the habit in the eyes of the public.

In stage three of the effort to control tobacco, Finland and Norway have both focused on nicotine as an addictive substance that can override good intentions to stop smoking. Although substitution treatments were tested by leading figures in Sweden in the 1950s (Elam, 2014), NRT gained serious traction in the 1990s and has since permeated much of the way in which the tobacco problem is conceived. In the 2010s, the e-cigarette is not only a substitute for nicotine ingestion, it also replicates the oral sucking sensation and the hand movements of the smoker.

In the 1970s, the smoker and the smoking habit were the target of interventions; in the 1980s, concern was for the 'side effects' of smoking; and in the

2000s, the question has been firmly anchored in the body and mind of the smoker. These conceptual positions and aspects of governance have been achieved by means of information, education, and legislation involving many different actors and stakeholders who have been willing to act on new knowledge and ideas. The history of tobacco control in Finland and Norway is by no means unique: in the Western world tobacco policy and control have followed the same chronological pattern—in parallel with new scientific advances.

References

Alasuutari, P., & Qadir, A. (2014). Epistemic governance: an approach to politics of policy-making. *European Journal of Cultural and Political Sociology*, **1**, 67–84.

Baglia, J., & Foster, E. (2014). 'Mad Men' as health communication: health-related themes in the hit AMC television series. *Health Communication* (early online).

Beck, C.J., Drori, G.S., & Meyer, J.W. (2012). World influences on human rights language in constitutions: a cross-national study. *International Sociology*, **27**(4), 483–501.

Bell, K. (2013). Tobacco control, harm reduction and the problem of pleasure. *Drugs and Alcohol Today*, **13**, 111–118.

Bell, K., Salmon, A., Bowers, M., Bell, J., & McCullough, L. (2010). Smoking, stigma and tobacco 'denormalization': further reflections on the use of stigma as a public health tool. *Social Science & Medicine*, **70**(6), 795–799.

Bell, K., & Keane, H. (2012). Nicotine control: e-cigarettes, smoking and addiction. *International Journal of Drug Policy*, **23**, 242–247.

Benowitz N.L. (1999). Nicotine addiction. *Primary Care: Clinics in Office Practice*, **26**(3), 611–631.

Berridge, V. (1998). Science and policy: the case of postwar British smoking policy. In S. Lock et al. (Eds.), Ashes to ashes: the history of smoking and health. Amsterdam: Rodopi. 143–162.

Berridge, V. (1999). Passive smoking and its pre-history in Britain: policy speaks to science? *Social Science & Medicine*, **49**(9), 1183–1195.

Bliksrud, T., & Nygaard, E. (2002). Røyketelefonen og endret røykeatferd [The smoke line and changing smoking behavior]. *Tidsskrift for Den norske legeforening*, **27**(122), 2616–2618.

Chapman, S. (2007). Public health advocacy and tobacco control: making smoking history. Oxford: Blackwell. Accessed 13 September 2014. http://samples.sainsburysebooks.co.uk/9780470691632_sample_382695.pdf

Chapman, S., & Freeman, B. (2008). Markers of the denormalisation of smoking and the tobacco industry. *Tobacco Control*, **17**(1), 25–31.

Cisneros Örnberg, J., & Sohlberg, T. (2012). Swedish Tobacco policy: from rational choice to 'harm to others'. In: Hellman, M., Roos, G., vonWright J. (2012). A Welfare Policy Patchwork: Negotiating the Public Good in Times of Transition. Helsinki: Nordic Center for Welfare and Social issues (NVC) pp. 65–82

Doll, R., & Hill, A. B. (1950). Smoking and carcinoma of the lung. *British Medical Journal*, **30**(2), 739–748.

Edwards, G. (1997). Alcohol policy and the public good. *Addiction*, **92**(s1), S73–S79.

Elam, M. (2012). Pharmaceutical incursion on cigarette smoking at the birth of the brain disease model of addiction. *Advances in Medical Sociology*, **14**, 53–75.

Elam, M. (2014). From the birth of the smokers' clinic to the invention of Nicorette: Problematizing smoking as addiction in Sweden 1955–1971. *Nordic Studies on Alcohol and Drugs*, **31**(5–6), 467–484.

Farsalinos, K.E., & Stimson, G. (2014). Is there any legal and scientific basis for classifying electronic cigarettes as medications. *International Journal of Drug Policy*, **25**, 340–345.

Glantz, S.E. (Ed.). (1996). The cigarette papers. Berkeley: University of California Press.

Glantz, S.E., & Balbach, E.D. (2000). Tobacco war: inside the California battles. Berkeley: University of California Press.

Hakkarainen, P. (2000). Tupakka—Nautinnosta ongelmaksi [Tobacco—from enjoyment to problem]. Tampere: Vastapaino.

Hakkarainen, P. (2013). Tobacco road Finland—how did an accepted pleasure turn into an avoidable risk behaviour? *Social Science & Medicine*, 98, 253–259.

Hallituksen Esitys (1993). HE 116/1993. Hallituksen esitys Eduskunnalle laiksi toimenpiteistä tupakoinnin vähentämiseksi annetun lain ja markkinatuomioistuimista annetun lain muuttamisesta [The government bill to the Parliament for changes in the Act about actions for reducing smoking and in the Act about Market Court].

Heloma, A. et al. (2012). Suomen tupakkapolitiikka ja lainsäädäntö—kehitys vuodesta 1976 nykypäivään [Tobacco policy and legislation in Finland from 1976 onwards]. In A. Heloma et al. (Eds.), Kohti savutonta Suomea [Towards tobacco-free Finland]. Helsinki: National Institute for Welfare and Health (THL). 24–35.

Helse- og omsorgsdepartementet (HOD). (2013). En framtid uten tobakk. Nasjonal strategi for arbeidet mot tobakksskader 2013–2016. Accessed 15 December 2015. http://www.regjeringen.no/upload/HOD/Dokumenter%20FHA/enfremtidutentobakk_nasjonalstrategi.pdf

Hoffman, A. L., & Slade, J. (1993). Following the pioneers: addressing tobacco in chemical dependency treatment. *Journal of Substance Abuse Treatment*, **10**(2), 153–160.

IPSA. (2014). Panel on Epistemic Governance. Accessed 15 December 2015. http://www.ipsa.org/my-ipsa/events/montreal2014/panel/epistemic-governance

Jackson, P. (1995). The development of a scientific fact: the case of passive smoking. In R. Bunton et al. (Eds.), The sociology of health promotion. London: Routledge. 103–115.

Joossens, L., & Raw, M. (2006). The Tobacco Control Scale: a new scale to measure country activity. *Tobacco Control*, **15**, 247–253.

Keane, H. (2002). Smoking, addiction and the making of time. In J.F. Brodie & M. Redfield (Eds.), High anxieties: cultural studies in addiction. Berkeley: University of California Press. 119–133.

Kinnunen, T., Korhonen, T., & Kaprio, J. (2012). Mitä uutta tupakkariippuvuudesta ja sen hoidosta? [What is new about tobacco addiction and treatment?] *Suomen Lääkärilehti*, **67**, 3559–3563.

Klein, A. (2013). Editorial: tobacco harm reduction—a new opportunity or a step too far? *Drugs and Alcohol Today*, **13**, 71–72.

Klein, R. (1993). Cigarettes are sublime. Durham, NC: Duke University Press.

Koo, J. W., & Ramirez, F. O. (2009). National incorporation of global human rights: worldwide expansion of national human rights institutions, 1966–2004. *Social Forces*, **87**(3), 1321–1353.

Leppo, K. (1978). Smoking control policy and legislation: letter from Finland. *British Medical Journal*, **1**, 345–347.

Lesmes, G.R., & Donofrio, K.H. (1992). Passive smoking: the medical and economic issues. *American Journal of Medicine*, **93**(1), S38–S42.

Lund, K.E. (2013). Hva er elektroniske sigaretter, hvor farlige er de og hvordan bør de reguleres? SIRUS-rapport. 5/2013.

McNeill A., et al. (2014). A critique of a WHO-commissioned report and associated article on electronic cigarettes. *Addiction*.

Meyer, J.W. (2008). Reflections on institutional theories of organizations. In R. Greenwood et al. (Eds.), The Sage handbook of organizational institutionalism. London: Sage. 790–811.

Norwegian Cancer Society (1967, April). Influencing smoking behaviour. Report from 'Utvalget for forskning i røykevaner' (the Bjartveit Committee), appointed by the Norwegian Cancer Society.

Örnberg, J.C. (2013). A solitary case: Swedish tobacco policy as harm reduction? *Drugs and Alcohol Today*, **13**(2), 102–110.

Piha, T. (1992). Fifteen years' experience of comprehensive tobacco control legislation. *Tobacco Control*, **1**, 239–240.

Proctor, R.N. (2012). The history of the discovery of the cigarette–lung cancer link: evidentiary traditions, corporate denial, global toll. *Tobacco Control*, **21**(2), 87–91.

Rimpelä, A. (1992). Critical analysis of the Finnish Tobacco Act: implementation and legitimacy, 1977–1989. *Tobacco Control*, **1**, 285–293.

Ruokolainen, O., Ollila, H., & Heloma, A. (2014). Sähkösavukkeiden käyttö Suomessa 2012 ja 2013 [Prevalence of electronic cigarettes in Finland 2012 and 2013]. Helsinki: THL, Tutkimuksesta tiiviisti.

Russell, M.A.H. (1976). Low-tar medium-nicotine cigarettes: a new approach to safer smoking. *British Medical Journal*, **1**, 1430–1433

Sæbø, G. (2012). The regulation of smoking and smokers in Norway 1964–2010. In M. Hellman et al. (Eds.), A welfare policy patchwork: negotiating the public good in times of transition. Helsinki: Nordic Centre for Welfare and Social Issues (NVC). 21–41.

Sæbø, G. (2014). Away with tobacco? on the early understandings of tobacco as a problem and the associated attempts at political regulation of tobacco in Norway 1900–1930. *Nordic Studies on Alcohol and Drugs*, **31**(5–6), 443–466.

Skretting, A., Lund, K.E. & Bye, E. (2014). Rusmidler i Norge 2013. Oslo: Statens institutt for rusmiddelforskning (SIRUS).

Royal College of Physicians. (1962). Smoking and health. A report of the Royal College of Physicians on smoking in relation to cancer of the lung and other diseases. London: Pitman Medical Publishing.

Stolerman, I.P., & Jarvis M.J. (1995). The scientific case that nicotine is addictive. *Psychopharmacology*, **117**(1), 2–10.

Sulkunen, P. (2009). The saturated society: governing risk and lifestyles in consumer society. London: Sage.

Tarnaala, E. (2005). Ehkäisevän päihdetyön käsitteestä. *Yhteiskuntapolitiikka-YP*, **70**(2), 188–196.

Thompson, L., Pearce, J., & Barnette, J.R. (2007). Moralising geographies: stigma, smoking islands and responsible subjects. *Area*, **39**(4), 508–517.

Tobacco Act. (1976). Act to reduce the harmful consequences of smoking. **693**. 13 August 1976.

Tobacco Act. (1994). Act about the reform of the act to reduce the harmful consequences of smoking. **765**. 19 August 1994.

Tobacco Act. (2010). Act about the reform of the act to reduce the harmful consequences of smoking. **698**. 20 August 2010.

Troyer, R. (1989). The surprising resurgence of the smoking problem. In J. Best (Ed.), Images of issues: typifying contemporary social problems. New York: Aldine de Gruyter. 159–176.

Tupakkariippuvuus ja tupakasta vieroitus. Käypä hoito suositus [Current care guideline: tobacco addiction and its cure]. 19 January 2012. Accessed 3 September 2014. http://www.kaypahoito.fi/web/kh/suositukset/naytaartikkeli/ . . . /hoi40020

U.S. Department of Health and Human Services (USDHHS). (1986). The health consequences of involuntary smoking: a report of the Surgeon General. http://profiles.nlm.nih.gov/NN/B/C/P/M/

U.S. Department of Health and Human Services (USDHHS). (1988). Nicotine addiction: the health consequences of smoking. A report of the Surgeon General. Accessed 8 December 2014 http://profiles.nlm.nih.gov/ps/access/NNBBZD.pdf.

Valverde, M. (1998). Diseases of the will: alcohol and the dilemmas of freedom. Cambridge, UK: Cambridge University Press.

West, R., & Grundberg, N. (1991). Editorial: implications of tobacco use as an addiction. *British Journal of Addiction*, **86**, 485–488.

WHO. (2013). WHO report on the global tobacco epidemic 2013: enforcing bans on tobacco advertising, promotion and sponsorship. Accessed 1 June 2015. http://www.who.int/tobacco/global_report/2013/en/

Wikipedia. (2014). Mad Men. Accessed 14 October 2014. http://en.wikipedia.org/wiki/Mad_Men

Wynder, E.L., & Graham, E.A. (1950). Tobacco smoking as a possible etiologic factor in bronchiogenic carcinoma; a study of 684 proved cases. *Journal of the American Medical Association*, **143**(4), 329–336.

Chapter 9

General practitioners' position on problematic gambling in three European welfare states

Michael Egerer, Matilda Hellman, Michał Bujalski, and Sara Rolando

9.1 The welfare cultural setting of general practitioners

General practitioners[1] (GPs) are at the forefront of professional medical practice. Their daily work typically involves dealing with the whole spectrum of medical problems in a rather tight time frame. Despite a well-established, evidence-based medical action repertoire, they constantly need to creatively apply their textbook knowledge to real-life medical problems in their practice (Abbott, 1988; Scott, 2008). This is especially true when facing conditions which are situated at the borders between physical, mental, and social matters and which are less clearly established as medical issues. But on what basis, if not on medical knowledge, will general practice then function?

Abbott (1988) describes professional (medical) practice as an endeavour of improvisation, where diagnosis and treatment often become one and the same. Professional knowledge also serves to secure a profession's turf. Freidson (1970) has suggested, on the other hand, that the authority of the medical profession cannot be based on its exclusive specialist knowledge alone, but rather on its deeply institutionalized position of power in the system of the bureaucratic nation state. He adds that the ways in which primary healthcare is arranged have a significant impact on the practice of GPs. For example, the doctor-patient relationship—generally considered a key for success in treatment—is influenced by circumstances such as frequency of meeting occasions, familiarity between physician and patient, and continuity of medical care—all of which have an influence on the physician's perception of patients and resolution of their problems (Baker, 1997; Freidson, 1970; Hakosalo, 2010; Hjortdahl, 1992; Kearley et al., 2001; Mayntz, 1970).

European comparisons, both with mass media materials and focus group interviews with welfare professionals (GPs and social workers), have shown that not only do the country-specific institutional arrangements of welfare service provision tend to colour the governing views on the problems, but also the country's traditional ways of addressing addiction-related problems will correlate with the present governing images of what addiction problems are all about (Egerer, 2014; Hellman et al., forthcoming).

The Finnish non-medical approach—placing reasons and consequences in the social realm—could be discovered in GPs' as well as social workers' discussions. The medical model, traditionally strong in France, came up in discussions of French professionals. Hellman and Room (2014) have demonstrated that the governing perception of how to help people with addiction problems is deeply embedded in the system's cultural characteristics. In Finland, with its rather individualistic universalist welfare culture, media reports on addiction tended to divide the responsibilities to solve addiction problems between the self-sufficient individual and the welfare state agents. In the U.S., on the other hand, meso-structures, like neighbourhood associations and church congregations, were pointed out as main actors to be involved for successfully solving the problems. Polish press material discusses addiction problems, similarly to Finland, more in social-political terms, whereas in Italy the family context seems most important (Beccaria et al., forthcoming; Hellman et al., forthcoming).

This chapter follows up the cultural embeddedness of medical expertise in three European countries by confronting medical practitioners with problem gambling—a problem that is not that directly ascribed to their professional field as is, for example, a broken leg or a clogged artery. In a situation without any clear evidence-based road maps for medical practitioners to use, we expect that the circumstances surrounding the routines and modes of practice of the profession will inevitably influence the ways in which the GPs deal with the question; and consequently will show up more clearly compared to looking at problems with a 'stronger . . . evidence of non-lingual symbols' (Spode 2005, p. 90; transl. M. Egerer), such as the already-mentioned broken leg or clogged artery. The role that is given to and taken by GPs as a profession is partly formed by the *welfare culture* of which it is part. A welfare culture consists of the country-specific bundles of values, ideas, and justifications concerning the promotion of welfare and the actors involved. The welfare arrangements of each of the studied countries—Finland, Italy, and Poland—are the sum of its country-specific welfare culture, social structures, actors, and institutions (Pfau-Effinger, 2005).

We study the dominating traits of argumentation in Finnish, Italian, and Polish GPs' discussions of problem gambling. On the basis of the discussions we try to situate their professional role towards the issue by paying special attention to the institutional setting of the profession in the welfare states under study. Studies of the involvement of GPs in handling problem gambling has been so far centred in Anglo-Saxon countries, hence in countries exemplifying a liberal arrangement of welfare institutions (Miller, 1996; Pasternak & Fleming, 1999; Sullivan et al., 1998). More recently the discussion about intervention in general practice for problem gambling has started also in other countries (Bellio & Fiorin, 2012; Capitanucci et al., 2006; Erbas B., Buchner, 2012; Komu et al., 2012). However, these take the institutional setting of GPs as given and lose the advantages of a cross-cultural comparison.

In this study we suggest that the framings of gambling problems found in our data sets from Finland, Italy, and Poland are not only the result of different cultures that 'inherently' have different views on problems and different ways of action in these matters. They also show footprints of each country's welfare culture, its arrangement of welfare institutions, and the common ways of approaching gambling and addiction problems. The traits of GPs' argumentation in the different countries will inevitably also be the result of the responsibilities given to the profession in its specific welfare state system. This assumption, although it might seem rather 'natural', in fact challenges both the basic idea of context-free, expert medical knowledge, as well as a simple medicalization theory limiting its scope to social control and the power endeavour of the medical profession (Rose, 2007; Ruuska, 2013). This study is part of the work package 'Images' of the Programme on Addiction and Lifestyles in Contemporary Europe: Reframing Addictions Project (ALICE RAP) funded by the European Union Framework Programme Seven (FP7). It aims at providing knowledge on how society defines, understands, and categorizes addictions.

9.2 **Cultural variations in the medical profession**

The healthcare and social services sectors grew and expanded with the rise of the welfare state in all Western societies from the 1920s to the 1980s. The systems evolved at different paces and in various modes, but the welfare state still remains the most common shape of democratic states. The rise of this statism involved an institutionalization of task divisions that came to coin definitions of attainable matters and the efforts for dealing with them. Historically, the notions of 'public health' and 'welfare of the people' have largely overlapped on the welfare state agenda.[2]

Applying the classic categorizations of welfare regimes (Esping-Andersen, 1990) to the countries under study, one can summarize that social democratic regimes with large public responsibility, like Finland, tend to organize their primary healthcare in centralized health centres. In Italy, a Southern subtype of the continental regime (Fenger, 2007), GPs instead mainly work in private practice. In contrast, Poland inherited a universal healthcare system on its way towards market economy in the 1990s, including occupational and school care. However, over the years these have been plagued by numerous problems, including corruption, inefficient management, and hierarchical structures with powerful physicians at the top and patients at the bottom.

9.2.1 **Finland**

Finnish primary healthcare is by municipalities. From the outset of the medical profession in Finland, doctors have been servants of the state sworn to the king (during the time Finland was a part of Sweden, 1150–1809) and later on to the Tsar (when part of Russia, 1809–1917). Physicians have been civil servants with an obligation towards the society as a whole. As part of the Finnish welfare state project, health centres were established in the 1970s, with doctors consisting mostly of GPs. This shift from the previous system of municipal doctors had a huge impact on professional autonomy and the doctor-patient relationship. In the new institutional setting, turnover of doctors became high. The doctor-patient relationship was limited temporally speaking; no long-term contacts could be established. Although efforts have been made to assign all citizens their 'own' nurses and GPs, these structural characteristics have remained in the Finnish primary healthcare system. The doctor-patient relationship in occupational health and municipality health centres, where most GPs are employed, can thus be viewed as a rather technical one, with a focus on bodily appearance, somatic symptoms, and adherence to pharmacological treatment. The diminishing doctor-patient relationship became an issue in the 1990s and a need for change was acknowledged. However, with the new era of the 'locum doctor', long-term relations between doctors and patients became even more difficult (Hakosalo, 2010).

Lately, occupational healthcare is increasingly supplementing basic primary healthcare, resulting in growing inequalities in service provision between those who are regularly employed and those who lack a stable continuous engagement in occupational life. Although services are more generous and quickly available, the organization of occupational healthcare is comparable to the municipal health centres; both resemble what Freidson (1970) identified as 'clinic organization'. Such an organization is inherently prone to disregarding the individual patient, failing to accommodate specific needs, and not considering the whole human being in its context. The advantage of easy availability of colleagues' support comes at the price of streamlining practice patterns and reinforcing institutional paradigms. Currently (2015) Finland is undergoing an extensive social and healthcare reform in which the aim is to integrate the social and healthcare sectors to the utmost extent possible (see Ministry of Social Affairs and Health, 2014). GPs are used to dealing with alcohol-related matters in their daily practice, although their role is comparable to doctors in war, who treat the wounded, but are not concerned about the reasons for the war itself (Takala & Lehto, 1988).

9.2.2 Italy

In Italy, the national health system was established in 1978 and inspired by solidarity principles. In 2000, by Law 328, the health and social systems converged into a unique system. Both the healthcare system and the social system were developed within the same perspective; namely, the assumption of the protection of the individual by the entire community. Social-health integration has been defined a strategic priority (DPR no. 23, 1998). However, this is not yet fully realized, as institutional, professional, and organizational gaps persist.

The primary healthcare system in Italy is formally based on the 'by initiative' paradigm oriented to 'active promotion' of health. It aims at strengthening personal (self-care and family learning) and social resources (proximity networks and social capital) available to the individual, especially those suffering from chronic diseases or disabilities. GPs are part of this system, having a special contract with the local health system in a position that can be seen as a mix of the role of a consultant and an employee. People can choose their own doctor, who is allowed to add clients until reaching a specified limit of patients (1,500).

A survey of GPs' attitudes towards assessment of pathological gambling (Capitanucci et al., 2006) has shown that in several cases clients spontaneously tell their problem to the practitioner. However, not many GPs actively ask questions aimed at individuating gambling problems, and around 40 per cent seem not to provide therapeutic interventions even when the problem has been identified. As the authors underline, among GPs there is a general uncertainness about their role on the matter; they are not properly trained to identify, assess, and provide medical care to clients with gambling problems. Indeed many GPs have said that their information sources are more frequently mass media than scientific articles.

A more recent study comes to similar conclusions, showing that about 25 per cent of GPs are scarcely aware of the problem; the GPs also seem reluctant to be involved in the treatment of the problem or in specific training (Bellio & Fiorin, 2012). The authors suggest that interventions most appropriate in the setting of general medicine seem to be screening and early detection, motivation and engagement, and monitoring. The same statement is reported in the *Manual for Professionals of Addiction* published by the Anti-Drug Policies Department (Serpelloni, 2013), where the importance of involving GPs is cited in relation to early identification of the problem and support for addicts and their families, along with a 'possible spiritual counsellor' (Serpelloni, 2013, p. 83; transl. S. Rolando) and other supporting figures in the social context. The reference to the religious sphere could sound odd, but the influence of the Catholic church in the definition and treatment of addiction problems has a long history in Italy. Before the development of public addiction services during the 1990s, heroin-addicted people were treated in therapeutic communities (TCs), run mostly by religious leaders who were against the medicalization of the problem and who strenuously promoted social rehabilitation and re-education as the solution (29). The mass media played a role in spreading the image of the addict as a moral sinner—in the early 1990s, still the most likely category (Beccaria et al., forthcoming). In the field of gambling the church has taken a clear position: in 2012 lay and Catholic non-profit organizations organized a massive national campaign to prohibit gambling advertising (Pedroni, 2014).

9.2.3 **Poland**

In Poland, the earlier-mentioned problems of primary healthcare of the 1990s were targeted with a large healthcare reform initiated late in the decade. The reform consisted of an application of market competition between healthcare providers from both the public and the private sector in order to enforce economic considerations within the system that had previously enjoyed permanent funding from the state budget. Special medical care taxes or dues were introduced to be paid by each employed citizen. The funds generated were supposed to be distributed by the independent public insurance body operating at the regional level initially called Kranken Kasses, which was, however, soon to be replaced by the more centralized National Health Fund (NHF), with branches across the country. Consumers were free to choose any facility for healthcare services; money from NHF followed the client who made the choice.

This seemingly rational market reform failed to be efficient. Patients tended to attend healthcare facilities which were the most attractive and which offered the most expensive treatment to be paid by the public insurance system. At the same time, other facilities, including large hospitals, became heavily indebted and found themselves on the verge of bankruptcy.

For these reasons, the market-based system of funding was replaced by a system of annual contracts between health providers, on the one hand, and the NHF, on the other. Health providers were paid according to number of services adopted in the contract, with notable exception of mental health services, which were paid by hospital person-days assumed to be necessary for different disorders. Another exception was primary healthcare, where GPs were paid by the number of patients who selected them as their own GP. As a result, a large arena for negotiations and pressures was established in which the power of corporate interests of different medical specializations dominated. The winners in this system were cardiology and oncology which were supposed to fight against the two biggest killers—heart disease and cancer—while mental health, including addiction treatment, was much less successful in fighting for public funds.

Another group that benefited were the GPs who had been able to recruit local corporations to negotiate their contracts. Such negotiations were prolonged as long as the NHF allowed access to GPs' services. Additionally, physicians in individual hospitals demanded increases in their salaries under threat of strike, including hunger strikes. Slowly, corporations of physicians, including the National Chamber of Physicians, grew to represent serious economic and political power in the public debate. As a rule, they represented traditional morals in a number of socio-medical questions, including their anti-abortion position, attempting to demonstrate their moral superiority and to justify their new economic gains. As a result, a highly hierarchical structure of power and management has been reinforced, and the weak position of patients—in particular, those with addiction problems—has been maintained.

9.3 Reception analytical group interviews

In Section 9.1, we presented the idea that GPs from the three countries under study would show differences in their views on gambling problems in line with, or due to, the welfare cultural context in which they perform their profession. In Section 9.2, we briefly described these contextual circumstances. Using a broad-brush approach, one can summarize as follows.

Finland has high-standard, highly accessible primary healthcare in line with the social democratic model. This system's weakness is its lack of personal interaction between a patient and the same doctor over time. The GP's practice thus tends to become a rather clinical, impersonal, diagnostically focused affair. On the other hand, Finnish GPs have a long tradition of encountering addiction problems, especially alcohol-related, in their daily praxis, and may be rather sensitive to these problems.

In Italy, the primary healthcare system has been based on the idea of activity and initiative on the clients' part. Medical doctors have shown limited interest in dealing with addiction-related matters; elderly doctors in particular have tended to internalize a view based on the re-educational stance of the Catholic church. Private lifestyle-related problems are to be dealt with in therapeutic communities or as a family matter.

In Poland, the recent history of primary healthcare is inscribed with trials and failures to apply market logic to the provision of healthcare services, based on the preferences of the patients. This has led to competitive stances both between GPs (relating to the number of patients who choose them), and between fields of expertise (radiology and oncology drawing the longest straw). The system, although corrected on many occasions, has tended to marginalize the fields of mental health and addiction problems.

In order to examine the argumentative traits in GPs' conceptualizations of problem gambling and relate these to their welfare cultural context, we performed reception analytical group interviews (RAGI; Sulkunen & Egerer, 2009). In focus-group settings, we showed three film clips depicting types of gambling problems[3] to stimulate a discussion in groups of GPs. In the first clip, from the motion picture *Owning Mahowny* (Kwietnowski, 2003), Dan Mahowny continues to gamble, although he already 'beat' the casino once. The second clip, from *Bord de mer* (Lopes-Curval, 2002), deals with an elderly lady, Rose, who, while winning the jackpot, promises her son to quit gambling. She nevertheless breaks the promise, continues to gamble, and ultimately loses her house. *Going for Broke* (Campbell, 2003) is the source of the third clip, which shows how Laura is so preoccupied with gambling that the fruit selection in the supermarket reminds her of slot-machine symbols. She interrupts her shopping and gambles at the slot-machine available in the shop. The three clips thus engage the topics loss of control, neglect of obligations, and cue dependency (Egerer, 2010).

The clips were always shown in the same order leaving the same time for discussion. Questions to orientate the discussion were listed on paper and distributed to the participants. However, participants were specifically instructed that these questions would be used to facilitate the discussion, but that they did not need to be answered during the discussions. Group discussions were self-led; the moderator intervened only if the discussion went too far off the topic. The video-recorded interviews were transcribed verbatim afterwards.

A total of thirty-five GPs participated in seven groups in Finland; forty-one in six groups in Italy; and forty-three in six groups in Poland. The majority of Finnish (66 per cent) and Polish (72 per cent) participants were female, whereas Italian participants were mainly male (71 per cent).

Following a grounded theory approach, we constructed our coding scheme beforehand (Strauss, 1987). We analyzed the interview material by using three basic categories:[4] reasons for, consequences of, and ways of addressing problem gambling. We differentiated the categories further to provide an overview of participants' argumentative traits. Using predefined codes limits the flexibility of our analysis. On the other hand, conducting the analysis in three different languages by three different research teams, we deemed this trade-off necessary to synchronize the organization of the interview material for our qualitative, in-depth analysis. Each coded 'case' is an uninterrupted meaning entity during the discussion. The length of these cases varies significantly.

We first surveyed the data quantitatively before proceeding with a qualitative analysis of the content (Becker, 1998; Silverman, 2001). The numeric overview of topics covered shows that in Poland, where gambling is a less common practice and not a topic of public debate, GPs discuss this issue less than they do in Finland and Italy (see Tables 9.1, 9.2, and 9.3). These overview tables are not to be considered as results in themselves, as the coding praxis varies between countries. Our main interest in this study is the ways in which GPs conceptualize problems. For this purpose the counting exercise might even be misleading: a question may be mentioned once, but in a way that gives it extra significance, whereas something that is normalized may not be mentioned at all, but in a hidden way permeate discussions. However, when checked against the meaning-based content of the interviews, we found that the tables did accurately portray the emphasis on different repertoires within which the GPs expressed their views and articulated their professional stances.

In the next sections, we account for some larger traits in the GPs' argumentation regarding reasons for and consequences of problem gambling, and ways in which they should be addressed.

Table 9.1 Reasons for problematic gambling: number of cases by country

REASONS	Finland	Italy	Poland
Biological	14 (0.12)	11 (0.08)	3 (0.09)
Psychological Emotion	28 (0.24)	8 (0.06)	11 (0.31)
Psychological Compulsion	26 (0.22)	25 (0.18)	5 (0.14)
Psychological Character	12 (0.10)	20 (0.15)	6 (0.17)
Social Macro	27 (0.23)	37 (0.27)	5 (0.14)
Social Micro	10 (0.09)	35 (0.26)	5 (0.14)
Total	**117**	**136**	**35**

Note. Numbers in parentheses indicate proportion of total cases.

Table 9.2 Consequences of problematic gambling: number of cases by country

CONSEQUENCES	Finland	Italy	Poland
Biological	8 (0.09)	10 (0.13)	2 (0.09)
Psychological	17 (0.19)	11 (0.14)	6 (0.27)
Social Person concerned	38 (0.42)	29 (0.36)	9 (0.41)
Social Environment	28 (0.31)	30 (0.38)	5 (0.23)
Total	**91**	**80**	**22**

Note. Numbers in parentheses indicate proportion of total cases.

Table 9.3 Ways of addressing problematic gambling: number of cases by country

Addressing the problem	Finland	Italy	Poland
Medical/Biological	10 (0.17)	27 (0.30)	2 (0.05)
Psychological Person concerned	12 (0.20)	17 (0.19)	11 (0.29)
Psychological Environment	7 (0.12)	3 (0.03)	5 (0.13)
Social Person concerned	6 (0.10)	6 (0.07)	1 (0.03)
Social Environment	24 (0.41)	37 (0.41)	19 (0.50)
Total	**59**	**90**	**38**

Note. Numbers in parentheses indicate proportion of total cases.

9.4 **Reasons for problem gambling**

We separated the explanatory reasons for problem gambling that were given by the GPs in the group discussions by using our predefined categories (see Table 9.1). Under biological reasons, we coded, for example, cases that were concerned with the role played by genes, endorphins, and neurobiological mechanisms in general. The category psychological emotion involves attributing the gambling activity to enjoyment and thrill-seeking by the problem gambler, but also the filling of a void with the gambling activity. Such a void was, for example, a boring family life or being in a relationship where one feels lonely nevertheless. Unexplained 'having to' and loss of control was coded under psychological compulsion. This category comes close to the general idea of Alcoholics (and Gamblers) Anonymous, as well as diagnostic tools which identify the excessive behaviour by a lost ability to stop gambling (or drinking) at will. Psychological character refers to cases that name psychological problems (often depression), which are compensated by inappropriate gambling behaviour.

Furthermore, nonpathological character traits, like extroversion, have been included under this category. Social reasons are separated between a macro dimension (e.g. the state, gambling providers, and media) and a micro dimension (family and peers).

Finnish participants often refer to circumstances in the psychosocial sphere. They do indeed also mention to some degree neurobiological mechanisms in order to make sense of excessive gambling, but their main discourse revolves around cognitive issues and inappropriate psychological compensating strategies, as in the following quotations concerning the clip from *Bord de mer*:

> I3: She got the jackpot and the thrill of ecstasy, yes, that she felt compelled to repeat this experience.
> I6: Yes. In fact I thought about it that the real thing is the way, not the goal, only how to get there, the win is nothing.
> I2: Yes, it is the notion of the coins starting to pour into the lap, and you want to hear it once more.
> I1: I came to think about human psychology, and one of the characters were so obsessed and depressed. This one feels more that it is a housewife who has lived a boring and depressing life and now dreams of anything that can make her life better.
> I2: Change.
> (Finnish GPs, Group 1)

The good feeling has to be repeated, although, as these quotations show, the participants do not necessarily agree whether it is the thrill of the win or gambling in general that will stimulate enjoyment. Still, gambling fulfils the function of an emotional regulator for problem gamblers.

In Poland, emotions were most often raised as a reason for gambling. The moment when coins flow out of a slot machine or the dice hit the table is referred to as great experiences for all players. But fun, thrills, and gaining the attention of people around may hide the progress of addiction behaviour. Aroused emotions distort rational thinking. Still, engaging in gambling is also a way to cope with the boredom and to spice up everyday life and in this way serves a function which can be rationally comprehended:

> I2: Maybe she has gone through weariness, boredom, and a well-rounded life before. She was a good mother, a good employee having high salaries, and then such an impulse as she wanted to feel the excitement, to try something else.
> (Polish GPs, Group 1)

This quote about the clip from *Going for Broke* is surprisingly similar to the Finnish GPs' conversation that was cited earlier, stimulated by the clip from *Bord de mer*. A 'strong character' is mentioned as a protective factor against problem gambling. Furthermore, gambling affordability is one of the major decisive questions that will affect the decision to gamble. In general, Polish GPs claim that gambling is available only for people with sufficient financial resources. However, lotto and scratch cards are forms of gambling designed for the wider public. The high density of sites offering easily accessible forms of gambling, such as slot machines, was recognized to be a purposeful action geared solely towards profit of the operators, and should be restricted by law. The reaction of the Finnish participants towards the clip—depicting a slot-machine inside a supermarket—was, however, quite different: Finnish GPs discussed the Finnish (quite liberal) gambling legislation as working to prevent gambling, in contrast to the situation in the U.S. shown in the clip from *Going for Broke*:

> I1: And it took the attention that the game was right beside the exit door. Yes, that way that you cannot pass without noticing it; that it is really beside it. There it of course draws her [to the game].
>
> I6: Yes, but in Finland they [the slot machines] are always at the other side of the cashier. In Finland she would have made it [without gambling].
>
> (Finnish GPs, Group 6)

Italian GPs place the origin of problem gambling in a psychosocial frame, but, in comparison to their Finnish and Polish colleagues, emphasized to a greater extent social factors, especially the family context. A recurrent theme is that the gambler may have had some lack of care during childhood which is not yet recovered. The family is seen as the real root problem of the addiction, before other subsequent and secondary factors. The social context, particularly the family in which a person has grown up, is identified as the origin of the problem; some kind of shortage is indicated. The same awareness of the context in the development of health problems was also found among Italian adolescents, in contrast to Finnish ones, who focus on personal shortcomings (Rolando & Katainen, 2014). This aspect—consistent with one aspect of collectivistic cultures; i.e. contextualism (Owe et al., 2013)—represents a divergence from the trend towards 'responsibilization' (Rose, 1996) which is more pronounced in more individualistic cultures.

> I4: To me [it] is particularly important the context, that is the social and family environment where these addictions originate. I think there are some shortcomings. At the end, this is somehow the conclusion of a situation, of a lack of something that has occurred before.
>
> (Italian GPs, Group 5)
>
> I7: What we have not discussed and it is not clear from the clips is what is behind these characters, that is the family where they originated [from]. Because very often they come from families already deviated.
>
> (Italian GPs, Group 2)

On the other hand, focus on the family can turn in a 'family responsibilisation'. Even when discussing the 'Balduzzi Decree' (2012) that forbade gambling near schools and places of worship, the idea of the family and the changes occurring to the family institution and its relationships is put forward as the reason for the increase in gambling. One participant seems to blame the fact that the State must regulate the gambling market just because families are not performing their role properly:

> I1: What I want to say is that family is lacking. Why we need to have a law to forbid gambling close to a school or a church? I wonder, where are the parents?
> I7: They aren't anymore.
> I1: If they are not anymore, then there is a lack
> I4: They would be working and taking turns in order to pay the IMU [a new tax on houses] [laughing].
> I3: But parents can't be there always and anyhow.
> I1: No, my parents were there.
> (Italian GPs, Group 4)

If gambling can be seen as rooted in family origins, it is also discussed as a possible escape from present family problems:

> I7: [The gambler] says: 'Shit! I have nothing in my family, I had a fight with my husband, with my kids; my kids drive me mad; I go gaming.'
> (Italian GPs, Group 5)

9.5 **Consequences of problem gambling**

Our coding scheme for the consequences of problem gambling differentiates between biological (somatic) problems, psychological issues, such as depression and suicide, and social consequences (for the problem gambler or people around; see Table 9.2). As biological consequences we coded, for example, when GPs were talking about the sweating gambler Dan Mahowny. Although suicide is indeed a biological consequence, we nevertheless coded statements mentioning gamblers' killing themselves as psychological; the psyche is here a significant intermediate step towards death through suicide. Social consequences not surprisingly include financial problems for the gamblers and their close ones, but also alienation and loneliness. It is obvious that categories overlap and that it is sometimes hard to distinguish reasons from consequences. On the other side, there were also clear cases, as when informants mentioned depression as an outcome of problem gambling.

When looking at the consequences of problem gambling, it seems that GPs from the three countries do not differ too much in their perception. The interviewees associate problem gambling with somatic consequences only sometimes. When they do, it is usually to compare health damage from substance-based addictions to gambling, which has at most minor health impairments like diarrhoea. The participants are instead clearly concerned with the negative social consequences for gamblers and their families:

> I3: And the experience that I have in my occupational healthcare practice, these problem gamblers, honestly, they frighten me. I have had some cases in my practice, but they have been in such an early stage that I sent them immediately to psychiatrist, to someone who knows how to handle those. Well, I know that I can do also something but still, it's awful if someone gambles the house of the family, the house of his/her kids. It's so terrible, so destructive.
>
> I1: Yes, and then in its own way, it is horribly insidious, as it [the problem gambling] does not show openly.
>
> (Finnish GPs, Group 2)

Polish GPs tended to focus more on the gambler's misery when discussing the loss of property, as well as alienation and losing social relationships in the first place, instead of the harm towards the family:

> I4: It's a loneliness.
>
> I3: They were both alone.
>
> I7. There was no one to give him a hand. To help somehow, to explain . . .
>
> (Polish GPs, Group 1)

The family plays a central role in the Italian welfare regime and it therefore comes as no surprise that the Italian participants also discussed the harm in the context of and towards the family. When participants think that gambling is often a result of old and new family problems, they also argue that causes and consequences are mixed, depicting a vicious circle:

> I7: I would also add that both alcoholism and gambling are like a cat chasing its tail. I mean, a vicious circle, because somebody jumps in these, in these dependencies because maybe something is missing in his family, because he or she lacks something, because s/he does not feel fulfilled, because s/he has no children and s/he jumps on these things, but sometimes it is the opposite. That is, sometimes it is just drinking or gaming that brings you to become a person without a job, without a family, without a personality . . . so I have to say that it is sometimes the cause, sometimes it's the effect of what you live every day.
>
> (Italian GPs, Group 5)

The gambler's neglect of responsibilities towards his/her family is in the view of participants the most difficult aspect to understand. This seems to be a behaviour so far away from the common values to be interpreted as a loss of the sense of reality. When the addict is seen as a perpetrator causing harms to relatives, as in the clip from *Bord de mer*, signs of moral judgement may emerge from discourses:

> I3: Yes, he lacks the sense of responsibility. And the same thing happens to the woman who gambles, she has lost the contact with the reality as well . . . then she gambles not only the won money, but also everything, even what she cared for so much.
> I5: Her son's legacy, the house.
> (Italian GPs, Group 6)

9.6 Addressing problem gambling

Ways of addressing problem gambling were coded in a way similar to our coding of consequences (see Table 9.3). Some discourse was categorized as medical/biological interventions, which includes talk about doctors' and health centres' possibilities of intervening in problem gambling. Psychological environment includes statements about psychiatry and psychological therapies and treatments. The category psychological person concerned subsumed talk about the willpower of gamblers to solve the problem themselves and the necessity of their voluntary participation in treatment. Similar to this category, but still significantly different, is social person concerned, which we used when GPs were discussing a self-induced change in lifestyle away from gambling, such as becoming religious or finding another significant hobby in life. Social environment is a rather broad category. It includes discussions about social work and state regulations, but also less institutionalized forms of help via the family, friends, or colleagues.

None of the GP groups in any country found that dealing with problem gambling was part of their remit. Participants sometimes even specifically state that problem gambling is not a medical matter:

> I4: Yes, is this a medical problem? Do we let them handle it themselves?
> I3: In my opinion this does not look at all like a medical problem.
> (Finnish GPs, Group 1)

Italian GPs gave many explanations about their powerlessness in addressing the problem. First, identifying the symptoms of gambling is very difficult, as there are no physical signs that a doctor could see and gamblers do not ask for help.

Moreover, GPs cannot do much for gamblers as they have no proper means to address problem gambling:

> I7: Maybe [for] the real addictions—cocaine, heroin . . . —the local services, the doctor, they can do much. On the contrary, for alcoholism and gambling is done less. Maybe because we have not instruments and ways to help these persons.
> (Italian GP, Group 5)

Lastly, Italian GPs do not feel they have the right to inquire and give moral suggestions to clients concerning their behaviours. This is a priest's role and potentially could be seen as an intrusion into family matters. From all these explanations, this conception of problem gambling is obviously farthest from that of a disease:

> I3: As a medical practitioner, I answer to the client's needs when the patient asks me, because I'm not a priest. I cannot tell him, 'Come on, don't do these things!' I mean, he would send me to hell, and he would ask, 'Who asked your opinion?' So I limit myself, if the patient asks me for help, then I intervene as a medical doctor, purely in the field of health. Especially since it is very difficult, or at least it seems to me, to intervene at family level, when you do not have all the [family] members' consent. So it is not that you can act as the Great Sage of the situations teaching lessons about life!
> (Italian GPs, Group 3)

The church as a moral actor was a factor that was non-existent in Finnish and Polish focus groups.

The perception of gambling among Polish GPs is narrow due to lack of knowledge and direct experience. It can be considered as a 'hidden' addiction and its 'invisibility' can be a serious barrier in access to treatment services. The problem with recognition of gambling addiction appeared in all focus groups. Gambling is much harder to identify than, for example, alcohol addiction:

> I8: We don't recognize the fact that people may have that [gambling] problem.
> (Polish GPs, Group 5)

Polish physicians claimed that they can see and feel those who abuse alcohol, as alcohol affects the body, which makes the addiction noticeable. Instead, our study's Polish participants claimed that gambling is a problem of a psychological nature:

> I7: It does not affect somatic health.
> (Polish GPs, Group 3)

However, to some extent a physiological mechanism is also acknowledged to be 'certainly the same' but 'less known so far'. The lack of knowledge on gambling issues creates a gap that must be filled with patients' initiative and motivation to treatment—they have to declare the fact of addiction by themselves. As one GP admitted,

> I4: We don't have the knowledge because these are people who do not confess to be gamblers.
> (Polish GPs, Group 5)

For GPs in all three countries, the psychiatrist or a psychologist is the expert who is able to treat problem gambling. This form of treatment, however, is seldom explained any further. Psychiatric (or psychological) treatment seems to be a 'black box' for the GPs. A much more discussed topic is the social environment and its possibilities in dealing with problem gambling. For Italian GPs, the social environment was the most frequently mentioned provider of help. This, however, does not necessarily mean that the GPs consider the family always as the best actor in handling problem gambling. Instead, we identified a more complex picture. The relatives are seen as crucial to the ability to overcome the problem, and accordingly, the lack of family is a predictor of failure.

> I2: Maybe the first help is to be by the family
> I5: Yes, when there is a family.
> I2: Indeed the housewife has done everything . . .
> I3: And surely people who are close to him.
> I2: Without family, alone, he can't do it.
> (Italian GPs, Group 6)

However, the role of relatives is often questioned because they are too involved and often play a collusive role with the gambler. For this reason, in the view of Italian GPs, they are also in need of help. Hence, either self-help groups open to the whole gambler's family or therapeutic communities, which imply a separation from the negative familial context, are seen to be the best solutions.

For the Polish GPs, the family is an important factor in handling problem gambling. The family was claimed to be the source of motivation and support for a gambler, which may facilitate the process of recovery from gambling addiction. Family is the first and most important witness to the problem because other people can be tricked or simply not know about the problem. Nevertheless, the support from other close contacts—friends or partners—may also play a vital role since they help to overcome the worst enemy of the addict—loneliness:

> I4: There must be a support from the family, because if there is no support and no agreement from a patient—there is nothing we can do.
> (Polish GP, Group 6)

Finnish GPs, in contrast, seem to have less trust in this 'meso structure of welfare provision' (Hellman & Room, 2014). In fact they discuss how the families in the film clips have failed in providing efficient help to the problem gambler. The Finnish informants instead demand that individual gamblers do their share in starting the recovery process. Through the reliance on the micro level of welfare provision, they are closer to the Polish GPs, who also believe in a strong character to prevent problem gambling. Then again, Polish and Italian participants criticized the state and gambling providers for not preventing problem gambling by limiting availability—a discourse which is much weaker in the Finnish discussions.

9.7 A welfare cultural framing of problem gambling

In this chapter we have explored GPs' conceptualizations of problem gambling in three different welfare contexts. A medical framing of problem gambling does not dominate any of the discussions. None of the participants perceived problem gambling as being an issue for their practice. The root and origin of the problem is discussed in psychosocial terms in all three countries. The negative consequences are perceived as even more similar as primarily contaminating the social world.

Under closer examination, it seems that the welfare context does have some impact on the GPs' positioning towards the problems. In Italy, the discourse of genesis and harm of problem gambling revolves around the contextual circumstances tied to family life, and a re-education model is often referred to. In Finland and Poland, on the other hand, gambling as an inappropriate emotional regulator is more discussed as a consequence of contemporary society and of individual problems. Participants from these two countries, however, differ significantly in their attitude towards gambling availability. Polish GPs were especially critical of their country's gambling legislation (although, in fact, availability of slot-machines especially is more restricted than in Finland). Finnish GPs in comparison seem to be content with their country's policy concerning gambling availability. The different context becomes most obvious when comparing the GPs' thoughts on how to address the problem. Whereas Finnish GPs tend to hold the individual responsible for solving the problem, they also rely on the welfare state to take responsibility for providing care for problem gamblers. In the context of a subsidiary welfare state, Italian and Polish GPs think that the family is an important actor in addressing problem gambling.

It seems that the historically grown, country-specific approaches to problems in general and the welfare culture shape the perspective of the GPs. On the one hand, Finnish GPs tend to replicate Nordic welfare states' inclusive all-embracing system logic, while, on the other hand, relying on some typical individual traits in the same culture (Hirschovits-Gerz et al., 2011), they expect individuals to use their own resources to recover. The Italian context of the Southern European welfare state regime (Ferrara, 1996) is especially articulated in GPs' discourse about familial relations and the social context. Here also the influence of the church in shaping the concept of addiction is made evident by references to priests and their possible 'jurisdiction'. The profound changes in Polish society associated with the introduction of a free market economy initiated deep changes in the perception of social problems, including their individualization. This also applies to gambling problems. Opinions of Polish GPs seem to lack a perspective on the general social structure: they see gambling as a psychological problem rather than social one. The problem arises from specific traits of individuals, either their psychological characteristics or life events, which are reinforced by easy access to gambling temptations.

The Finnish GPs tended to apply a non-medical (social) frame to the problem; they did not object to the present rather liberal gambling legislation. They claimed a specific role in the Finnish welfare state and denied responsibility for treating problem gambling. Italian GPs often referred to the 'drug-based' addiction treatment as a reference point; they were rather critical of the recent liberalized gambling regulation. The Polish GPs also saw that gambling availability needs to be limited. In particular, slot-machine accessibility was pointed out as problematic; banning these machines outside casinos was seen as a way to control gambling activities. Similar to their Finnish colleagues, Polish GPs did not perceive gambling treatment as their responsibility. Instead, they tended to pay more attention to the role of the family and to the personal attributes of a gambler in the process of recovery. Abstracting these findings by grouping the suggested help provision according to their context of scale (see Hellman & Room, 2014), it seems that Finnish GPs put an emphasis on either the micro (individual responsible) or the macro context (welfare state level). The Italian participants, on their part, tended to value the meso level context (family or communities), whereas Polish physicians referred especially to micro (individual) and meso (family) settings.

The ways in which the GPs in the three countries speak about problem gambling as a matter to be dealt with follows to some extent some characteristic traits of the general welfare culture of which they are part. Naturally, within the frame of our study design we have no precise knowledge of the ideas that the participants from the different countries would attach to concepts like 'family' or 'therapy'. Italian and Polish participants seemed, for example, to include close friends in the family concept. This is important to keep in mind, for example, when drawing conclusions concerning the role of the family in dealing with the problem. Nevertheless, this circumstance does not render our categorization of the levels of addressing the problems—micro, meso, macro—of the welfare provision as misleading. In Table 9.4 we have summarized the circumstances in the welfare cultures that we see as scaffolding some typical conceptualizations in the GPs' discussions of problem gambling.

Our study points out the flaws in the idea of a transnational, objective medicine. The medical profession is not globally uniform; medical knowledge and especially practice differs from country to country (e.g. DeVries et al., 2001; Kleinman, 1980). The evolution of the profession is connected to deep cultural structures and dispositions of help provision. Our study has shown that it is essential to look also at the organization of (primary) healthcare, as well as at institutionalized practices of help, in order to understand how GPs see their role in addressing problem gambling. These findings also question the notions of a simple medicalization of former social problems. Instead they point to a more complex picture, where institutional structures and routines have an influence on how problems are perceived.

In the future, GPs might become obliged to increasingly deal with gambling problems in their day-to-day work. As in the case of alcohol (e.g. Fleming et al., 1997), brief interventions could be an efficient form to address problem gambling in the future; indeed this has already been suggested on many occasions (see e.g. Christensen et al., 2001; Miller, 1996; Pasternak & Fleming, 1999; Sullivan et al., 1998).

However, looking at the results of our study in the context of the Finnish, Italian, and Polish welfare arrangements, GPs might not be the right group to do so. Implementation would not only mean extensive training of the practitioners, but also require a considerable amount of adjustment in GPs' contexts. In a recent 'sister study' on Finnish and French social workers, Egerer (2013) showed that Finnish social workers seem to some extent comfortable with the role of dealing with problem gambling. This would perhaps render an implementation of brief interventions into social work offices, at least in Finland, feasible.

The results of this study also point out some challenges for any attempt to standardize and mainstream the medical profession in a multicultural context such as

Table 9.4 General welfare context and GPs' conceptualizations by country

	Finland	Italy	Poland
Welfare culture	Individualism & universalism	Family & church, active help-seeking	Social market economy & individualism
Welfare system: organization of primary healthcare	Social democratic: health centre & specialized general practice	Southern European/ continental: GPs mainly in private offices under contract with public healthcare	continental/'emergency welfare state': primary healthcare system has a near history of marketization
Gambling legislation and culture	monopoly & wide availability & positive image	licence-based system & recent heavy increase in availability	licence-based system, wide availability of lotto and slot machine gambling
Traditional way of addressing addiction problems	non-medical & alcohol & social work	moral & therapeutic communities & drugs & nonpharmacological	medical & social for alcohol; therapeutic communities for drugs
GPs' conceptualization: **reasons, consequences, and addressing problem gambling**	psychological/ cognitive frame, emotional regulator;	family dysfunction;	psychological/cognitive frame, emotional regulator, but also too low level of state control;
	negative social consequences;	negative social consequences;	negative individual and social consequences;
	not issue for GPs, instead individual & psychiatrist	not issue for GPs, instead family & community	not issue for GPs, instead family & individual & alternatively psychological treatment

the European continent. Actors involved in standardization of help provision and/or the education of professions need to look at the whole context of the professions concerned. Professions are integrated into the full network of welfare arrangements in which the various components interact with and depend on each other. Tinkering with only one component might not lead to the desired results.

Notes

1 General practitioners, or medical practitioners, are physicians who are at the front line of medical practice. They normally are the first physicians that patients see when having a medical problem.

2 The translation of such aggregate-level credos into normative arguments concerning the lifestyle choices of individuals has become increasingly challenging, as the welfare state project itself has facilitated citizens' autonomy, their rights, and potential to choose a preferred way of living (Sulkunen, 2009).

3 The original study involved also clips about problem drinking and eating (Egerer, 2014)

4 In order to organize the coding we used Atlas.ti (Finland and Italy) and Nvivo 7 (Poland) QDA software. Each team independently analyzed the transcripts in the original language, but used the same coding categories.

References

Abbott, A. (1988). The system of professions: an essay on the division of expert labor. Chicago: University of Chicago Press.

Baker, R. (1997). Will the future GP remain a personal doctor? *British Journal of General Practice*, **47**(December), 831–834.

Beccaria, F., & Rolando, S. (2013). Stakeholders' role in contemporary 'substitute drug' prescribing policies in Italy. *Substance Use & Misuse*, **21**(4), 387–405.

Beccaria, F., Rolando, S., Hellman, M., Bujalski, M., & Lemmens, P. (forthcoming). From criminals to celebrities: perceptions of 'the addict' in the print press from four European countries. *Substance Use & Misuse.*

Becker, H. (1998). Tricks of the trade: how to think about your research while doing it. Chicago: University of Chicago Press.

Bellio, G., & Fiorin, A. (2012). Gioco d'azzardo patologico: quale ruolo per il medico di medicina generale? [Pathological gambling: what role for the general practitioner?]. *Italian Journal on Addiction*, **2**(3–4), 121–127.

Campbell, G. (director). (2003). Going for broke [motion picture].

Capitanucci, D., Smaniotto, R., Biganzoli, A., Capelli, M., Alippi, M., & Fantoni, M. (2006). Indagine sulle attitudini di assessment del gioco d'azzardo patologico in un campione di medici di medicina generale e pediatri di libera scelta. [Research on the attitude towards assessment of pathological gambling in a sample of general practitioners and paediatricians]. *Società Italiana di Medicina Generale*, **3**, 7–9.

Christensen, M., Patsdaughter, C., & Babington, L. (2001). Health care providers' experiences with problem gamblers. *Journal of Gambling Studies*, **17**(1), 71–79.

DeVries, R., Benoit, C., van Teijlingen, E., & Wrede, S. (Eds.). (2001). Birth by design: pregnancy, maternity care, and midwifery in North America and Europe. New York: Routledge.

Egerer, M. (2010). Gate keepers' images of addiction in Finland, France, and Germany. The film-clips in the group interviews. Helsinki: University of Helsinki, Department of Social Research.

Egerer, M. (2013). Problem drinking, gambling and eating—three problems, one understanding? a qualitative comparison between French and Finnish social workers. *Nordic Studies on Alcohol and Drugs*, **1-2**, 67–86.

Egerer, M. (2014). Institutional footprints in the addiction image: a focus-group study with Finnish and French general practitioners and social workers [doctoral dissertation]. ed. Helsinki: University of Helsinki.

Erbas, B., & Buchner, U. (2012). Pathologisches Glücksspielen. Prävalenz, Komorbidität, Diagnose und Hilfsangebote in Deutschland. [Pathological gambling. Prevalence, comorbidity, diagnosis and support services]. *Deutsches Ärzteblatt*, **109**(10), 173–180.

Esping-Andersen, G. (1990). The three worlds of welfare capitalism. Cambridge: Polity Press.

Fenger, H. (2007). Welfare regimes in Central and Eastern Europe: Incorporating post-communist countries in a welfare regime typology. *Contemporary Issues and Ideas in Social Sciences*, **3**(2), 1–30.

Ferrara, M. (1996). The 'southern model' of welfare in social Europe. *Journal of European Social Policy*, **6**, 179–189.

Fleming, M.F., Barry, K.L., Manwell, L.B., Johnson, K., & London, R. (1997). Brief physician advice for problem alcohol drinkers: a randomized controlled trial in community-based primary care practices. *Journal of the American Medical Association*, **277**(13), 1039–1045.

Freidson, E. (1970). Professional dominance: the social structure of medical care. New Brunswick: Aldine Transaction.

Hakosalo, H. (2010). Katsaus lääkäriprofession kehitykseen Suomessa. Lääkäri, yhteiskunta ja yhteisö. [Overview of the development of the medical profession in Finland. Physician, society and community]. *Duodecim*, **126**, 1544–1551.

Hellman, M., Majamäki, M., Rolando, S., Bujalski, M., & Lemmens, P. (forthcoming). What causes addiction problems? environmental, biological and constitutional explanations in press portrayals from four European welfare societies. *Substance Use & Misuse.*

Hellman, M., & Room, R. (2014). What's the story on addiction? popular myths in the USA and Finland. *Critical Public Health*. doi: 10.1080/09581596.2014.926308

Hirschovits-Gerz, T., Holma, K., Koski-Jännes, A., Raitasalo, K., Blomqvist, J., Cunningham, J., et al. (2011). Is there something peculiar about Finnish views on alcohol addiction? a cross-cultural comparison between four northern populations. *Research on Finnish Society*, **4**, 41–54.

Hjortdahl, P. (1992). The influence of general practitioners' knowledge about their patients on the clinical decision-making process. *Scandinavian Journal of Primary Health Care*, **10**(4), 290–294.

Kearley, K., Freeman, G., & Heath, A. (2001). An exploration of the value of the personal doctor-patient relationship in general practice. *British Journal of General Practice*, **51**, 712–718.

Kleinman, A. (1980). Patients and healers in the context of culture. An exploration of the borderland between anthropology, medicine, and psychiatry. Berkeley: University of California Press.

Komu, I., Pajula, M., Kämppi, J., & Bergroth, M. (2012). Rahapelaaminen ja peliongelma. Lyhyesti ja selkeästi. [Gambling and gambling problems. Brief and clear]. Helsinki: THL.

Kwietnowski, R. (director). (2003). Owning Mahowny [motion picture]. Canada.

Lopes-Curval, J. (director). (2002). Bord de mer [Seaside; motion picture].

Mayntz, R. (1970). The nature and genesis of impersonality: some results of a study on the doctor-patient relationship. *Social Research*, **37**, 428–446.

Miller, M. (1996). Medical approaches to gambling issues—I: the medical condition. *Wisconsins Medical Journal*, **95**(9), 623–634.

Ministry of Social Affairs and Health. (2014). Social welfare and health care reform. Accessed 27 June 2014. http://www.stm.fi/en/ministry/strategies/service_structures

Owe, E., Vignoles, V.L., Becker, M., Brown, R., Smith, P.B., Lee, S.W., et al. (2013). Contextualism as an important facet of individualism collectivism: personhood beliefs across 37 national groups. *Journal of Cross-Cultural Psychology*, **44**(1), 24–45.

Pasternak, A., & Fleming, M. (1999). Prevalence of gambling disorders in a primary care setting. *Archives of Family Medicine*, **8**(6), 515–520.

Pedroni, M. (2014). The 'banker' state and the 'responsible' enterprises: capital conversion strategies in the field of public legal gambling. *Rassegna Italiana di Sociologia*, **55**(1), 71–98.

Pfau-Effinger, B. (2005). Culture and welfare state policies: reflections on a complex interrelation. *Journal of Social Policy*, **34**(1), 3–20.

Rolando, S., & Katainen, A. (2014). Images of alcoholism among adolescent in individualistic and collectivistic geographies. *Nordic Studies on Alcohol and Drugs*, **31**(2), 1–17.

Rose, N. (1996). Governing 'advanced' liberal democracies. In A. Barry et al. (Eds.), Foucault and political reason: liberalism, neo-liberalism, and rationalities of government. Chicago: University of Chicago Press. 327–356.

Rose, N. (2007). Beyond medicalization. *Lancet*, **369**, 700–702.

Ruuska, A. (2013). Consequences and behaviour problematised: the establishment of alcohol misuse as an object of empirical inquiry in late 18th- and early 19th-century European medicine. *Nordic Studies on Alcohol and Drugs*, **30**(1–2), 13–32.

Scott, R. (2008). Lords of the dance: professionals as institutional agents. *Organization Studies*, **29**, 219–238.

Serpelloni, G. (2013). Gambling. Manuale per i Dipartimenti delle Dipendenze.

Silverman, D. (2001). Interpreting qualitative data: methods for analyzing talk, text and interaction (2nd ed.). London: Sage.

Spode, H. (2005). Was ist Alkoholismus? Die Trunksucht in historisch-wissenssoziologischer Perspektive. [What is alcoholism? The drinking disease under the perspective of historical sociology and sociology of knowledge]. In B. Dollinger & W. Schneider (Eds.), Sucht als Prozess. Sozialwissenschaftliche Perspektiven für Forschung und Praxis. Berlin: VWB. 89–121.

Strauss, A. (1987). Qualitative analysis for social scientists. Cambridge: Cambridge University Press.

Sulkunen, P., & Egerer, M. (2009). Reception analytical group interview: a short introduction and manual. Helsinki: University of Helsinki, Department of Sociology.

Sulkunen, P. (2009). The saturated society: governing risk and lifestyles in consumer culture. Thousand Oaks, CA: Sage.

Sullivan, S., Arroll, B., Coster, G., & Abbott, M. (1998). Problem gamblers: a challenge for GPs. *NZ Family Physician*, **25**(1), 37–42.

Takala, J., & Lehto, J. (1988). Suomen alkoholihoidon kehitys ja ei-medisiininen malli. [The development of the Finnish alcohol treatment and the non-medical model]. *Sosiaalipolitiikka*, **13**: 105–125.

Chapter 10

Popular images of addiction in five European countries

Jan Blomqvist, Kirsimarja Raitasalo, Hans Olav Melberg, Dirk Schreckenberg, Christine Peschel, Justyna Klingemann, and Anja Koski-Jännes

10.1 Popular images of addiction

Mind-altering substances have been used throughout human history. However, which substances have been preferred and socially accepted, and which have been condemned and combatted, has varied with cultures and historical times (Blomqvist, 2004). Indeed, there are indications that the extent to which someone's substance use is likely to get them into difficulties, and evolve into what is regarded as an 'abuse' or an 'addiction', may not only depend on the pharmacological properties of the drug in question, or the neuropsychological characteristics of the user, but also to a large extent on the reactions with which the user is met, by the environment and by society at large (Blomqvist, 2004). For example, prevailing views that stigmatize a certain use may prevent people from seeking help for substance-related problems, imply cheaper or less effective help alternatives if they do, and/or lead to discrimination in work life or other life areas of addicts or ex-addicts (Blomqvist, 2012). Ideas about the unchangeable character of various kinds of substance use problems or addictions may hamper the environment's inclination to provide help and support, as well as the problem users' confidence in their own ability to find a solution (Blomqvist, 2002; Klingemann, 1992). In this way, addiction can be seen as 'interactive' in its essence, i.e. as a phenomenon, the official and predominant definition of which influences the self-definitions and behaviours of those defined, thereby serving, to an extent, as a self-fulfilling prophecy (Hacking, 1999).

In spite of the potentially vast consequences of such culturally dominant 'governing images' (Room, 1978) or 'social representations' (Moscovici, 1981, 1988) of various forms of substance use problems, our knowledge of how these vary between various forms of substance use and various cultural or geopolitical contexts is far from comprehensive. Trying to fill this knowledge gap can be considered an important task, not least at a time when addiction is increasingly seen as a global phenomenon (Alexander, 2008). The recent decade has also seen some efforts to fulfil at least part of this task. Examples are the Swedish research project 'The Social Context of Recovery—Views of Addiction and Recovery in the Population and in Various Professional Groups' (Blomqvist, 2009, 2012; Samuelsson et al., 2013), which explored Swedish lay and professional respondents' images of nine different addictions. In an expansion of this study comparable investigations have been conducted in Finland, Canada, and to some extent Russia (Cunningham et al., 2012; Holma et al., 2009; Koski-Jännes et al., 2012). As part of a further expansion of this investigation, similar studies have later been conducted in Poland, Norway, and Germany, meaning that there are now comparable data on the dominant popular images of addiction from five European countries. Available data enable the investigation of differences in the general public's images of nine different addictions[1] as well as cross-cultural variations in this respect.

10.2 **Study proceedings**

The study builds on previous research about how various addictions are perceived by lay people in different countries. More specifically, the study takes its point of departure in the previously mentioned Swedish survey, where a representative population sample, as well as representative samples of addiction treatment professionals were asked about their perceptions, in a number of different aspects, of nine different addictions (Blomqvist, 2009; Samuelsson et al., 2013). The original data for this survey were gathered in 2005—2006. About one year later, the study was replicated in Finland, Canada, and parts of Russia, within the framework of the international collaborative framework Images and Theories of Addictive Behaviours (http://blogs.helsinki.fi/imagesofaddiction/). Results from the Finnish and Canadian studies have previously been presented in separate articles (Cunningham et al., 2012; Cunningham et al., 1998; Holma et al., 2009; Koski-Jännes et al., 2012). The original Swedish survey, as well as the Finnish replication, were conducted as postal surveys, directed to random census samples, whereas the Canadian study was conducted as a telephone interview, performed by random digit dialling. The Finnish survey was, in applicable parts, a direct translation of the Swedish survey, whereas the script for the Canadian computer-assisted interviews (CATI) required some adaptions of the questionnaire to secure validity and comparability. These changes were agreed between responsible researchers in the three countries involved.

As part of the EU-funded ALICE RAP project,[2] similar studies were later conducted in Norway, Poland, and Germany. For economic reasons these studies were limited to a number of 'core questions' to ensure compatibility between countries. More specifically, the questions asked how respondents perceived the social severity of various addictions; the addictiveness of various substances or behaviours; the responsibility for acquiring and solving various addictions; and the options for recovering from various addictions, with or without formal treatment. In addition, it was decided that participants would, for convenience reasons, have the option of including these core questions within larger, ongoing, or planned omnibus surveys or investigations. Further, it was agreed that partners would have the option of adding other addictions than those that were included in the original Swedish study, if they were thought to be of particular national interest. The final core questions and their wording in English, in a survey version, were decided at a meeting between the partners in 2012, and further checked and corrected through mail discussions during the autumn of 2012. The Canadian telephone interview version was offered as a basis for formulating interview questions for partners who preferred this mode of data collection.

The data collection took place in 2005–2006 (Sweden), 2007 (Finland), 2012 (Norway), and 2013 (Poland and Germany). In total, almost 5,000 respondents were approached; response rates varied between 37 per cent (Finland) and 54 per cent (Sweden). To compensate for attrition bias, data were weighted for age and gender (all countries), education (Sweden and Norway), and marital status, income, and country of origin (Sweden only). All analyses are based on weighted data, whereas sample sizes rely on un-weighted data. The study characteristics are summarized in Table 10.1. As discussed Section 10.4.1, even if measures

Table 10.1 Summary of Study Characteristics

Country	Poland	Norway	Germany	Finland	Sweden	All
Sampling	RDD	RWP	RDD	RCS	RCS	
N	1000	1002	1003	740	1098	4843
Part of larger study	Yes	Yes	No	No	No	
Response rate	n a	52%	52%	37%	54%	
Year of data collection	2013	2012	2013	2007	2005/6	
Calibration variables	age, gender	age, gender, education	age, gender	age, gender	age, gender, marital status, income, country of origin	

RDD = Random digit dial; RWP = Representative web panel; RCS = Random census sample.

Table 10.2 Respondents' sociodemographics

Country	Poland	Norway	Germany	Finland	Sweden	All	p-value
Women (%)	50.6	50.5	51.7	51.3	49.6	50.7	ns
Age (SD)	42.0 (14)	47.2 (17)	49.5 (17)	45.6 (15)	44.2 (15)	45.7 (16)	< 0.001[a]
University educated (%)	21.4	32.8	30.4	27.5	32.9	29.3	< 0.001

Scheffé post hoc tests*: [a]G > N, F > S; P.

*Scheffé post hoc tests have been used throughout the analyses to explore homogenous subsets of countries.

Table 10.3 Respondents' substance use experiences

Country	Poland	Norway	Germany	Finland	Sweden	All	p-value
Substance							
Alcohol use (%)							
Current	89.2	n a	84.4	88.2	87.7	87.3	< 0.001
Previous	8.7		3.9	8.1	6.3	6.7	
Cannabis use (%)							
Current	2.8	n a	3.1	4.2	1.7	2.9	< 0.01
Previous	7.8		14.7	12.4	13.8	12.2	
Med. drugs (illegal use; %)							
Current	6.5	n a	2.6	6.1	1.8	4.1	< 0.001
Previous	5.2		1.4	4.9	3.1	3.6	
Smoking (%)							
Currently	23.0	n a	n a	20.4	20.6	21.4	n s
Previous	24.3			21.9	22.3	22.9	
Ever 'hard' drug use (%)							
Heroin	0.5	n a	0.8	1.1	0.7	0.7	n s
Amphetamines	2.7	n a	3.0	3.2	4.6	3.4	< 0.001
Cocaine	0.6	n a	2.5	1.7	2.5	1.9	< 0.01
Other 'hard' drugs	n a	n a	n a	4.3	n a	n a	

*Since data were collected at different points in time in different countries, any conclusions with regard to the representativeness of the national samples need to be drawn with caution.

were taken to prevent various forms of bias, the fact that national data were collected at different points in time and with different data collection methods warrants caution in interpreting the results.

Table 10.2 shows the gender, age, and highest education of those who responded to the questions in different countries. As concerns the latter variable, and due to differences in the national school systems, only the proportions with university education are shown. As can be seen, 50.7 per cent of the respondents were women (no significant differences between countries), and the mean age was 45.7 years, with Germans significantly older, and Poles and Swedes significantly younger, than Finns and Norwegians. Between less than one fourth (Poland) and almost one third (Sweden) of the respondents were university educated. However, it needs to be underlined that the differences between the five countries in this respect may partly be due to differences with regard to how university education is officially delimited, and this result should probably be taken with a grain of salt (cf. the previously mentioned caution).

Table 10.3 shows respondents' personal substance use experiences which may to some extent have influenced their perceptions of various addiction problems (Blomqvist, 2012; Cunningham et al., 2012).

10.3 **Perceptions of addiction**

The aim of the analyses has been to uncover how lay people from five European countries (Poland, Norway, Germany, Finland, and Sweden) perceive the severity of addictions as well as the individual risk of being afflicted by these addictions, and the probability of recovering from the same problems, with and without professional help. In addition, the aim was to explore attributions of responsibility for acquiring and desisting from these problems. A further aim has been to explore differences between the five countries.

10.3.1 **The perceived social severity of various substances and activities**

Table 10.4 shows how respondents rated the severity of various addictions as social problems. It should be observed that this question did not include addiction to Internet use, and that addictions to amphetamines, cocaine, and heroin were here lumped together as addiction to 'hard' drugs.

As shown in the table, addiction to 'hard' drugs is overall perceived as the most serious addictive problem to society, and gambling as the least severe problem. However, there are interesting between-country differences.

Table 10.4 Perceived social severity of various addictions (not at all serious = 1, extremely serious = 10)

Country	Poland	Norway	Germany	Finland	Sweden	All	p-value
Addiction to							
'Hard' drugs	7.84 (2.5)	8.38 (1.8)	7.15 (2.1)	7.43 (2.2)	8.66 (1.9)	7.93 (2.2)	< 0.001[a]
Alcohol	8.00 (2.14)	7.57 (2.02)	7.19 (2.0)	7.65 (2.0)	7.61 (2.2)	7.60 (2.1)	< 0.001[b]
Cannabis	7.45 (2.7)	7.00 (2.5)	6.18 (2.5)	6.66 (2.6)	8.15 (2.3)	7.13 (2.6)	< 0.001[c]
Medical Drugs	5.83 (2.4)	6.99 (2.1)	6.15 (2.3)	6.17 (2.2)	7.33 (2.4)	6.52 (2.4)	< 0.001[d]
Tobacco	7.14 (2.4)	5.56 (2.3)	5.91 (2.3)	6.37 (2.2)	5.75 (2.5)	6.13 (2.4)	< 0.001[e]
Gambling	6.14 (2.6)	5.97 (2.4)	5.94 (2.3)	5.15 (2.4)	6.44 (2.5)	5.97 (2.5)	< 0.001[f]
Overall	*7.07 (1.8)*	*6.90 (1.6)*	*6.43 (1.7)*	*6.56 (1.7)*	*7.32 (1.8)*	*6.88 (1.8)*	*< 0.001[g]*

Scheffé post hoc tests: [a]S, N > P, G > F, G; [b]P > F, S, N > G; [c]S > P > N, F > G; [d]S > N > F, G > P; [e]P > F > G > S, N; [f]S > P > N, G > F; [g]S > N > F, G.

Poles, Germans and Finns perceive addiction to alcohol as the addiction problem that is most serious to society, whereas Swedes and Norwegians reserve this place for addiction to 'hard' drugs. At the other end of the scale, Swedes and Norwegians perceive the use of tobacco as the least severe of the six mentioned addictions, whereas Poles allot that place to illegal use of medical drugs, and Finns to gambling. Notably, Swedes rate addictions to 'hard' drugs and cannabis as significantly more serious to society than respondents from any of the other countries do. At the same time they, together with Norwegians, see tobacco use as less serious than all other respondents. Finally, Swedes seem overall to rate addiction problems as more serious to society, and Germans and Finns as less serious, than others do.

To put addiction problems somewhat in perspective, Table 10.5 compares respondents' ratings of the severity of these problems with how they rated the severity of a number of other social problems. In this table data for addictions to Internet use are missing, and addiction to 'hard' drugs refers to addictions to amphetamines, cocaine, and/or heroin.

As the table shows, violent crime (defined as lethal or very severe violence) is seen as the most severe of the rated problems by respondents in all countries but Poland, where poverty is judged as an even more serious problem. Overall, however, addictions seem to be rated lower in severity

Table 10.5 Perceived severity of substance use problems and some other social problems in rank order

Rank	Poland	Norway	Germany	Sweden	Finland	All
1	Poverty	Violent crime	Violent crime	Violent crime	Violent crime	Violent crime
2	Violent crime	*'Hard' drugs*	Poverty	*'Hard' drugs*	*Alcohol*	*'Hard' drugs*
3	Environment	Theft	*Alcohol*	Environment	*'Hard' drugs*	Poverty
4	*Alcohol*	*Alcohol*	*'Hard' drugs*	Theft	Environment	Theft
5	*'Hard' drugs*	Poverty	Theft	*Cannabis*	Theft	Environment
6	Finance crime	Finance crime	Environment	Finance crime	Finance crime	*Alcohol*
7	Wage diff.	*Cannabis*	Wage diff.	Poverty	*Cannabis*	Finance crime
8	Theft	*Medical drugs*	Finance crime	*Alcohol*	Poverty	*Cannabis*
9	*Cannabis*	Environment	*Cannabis*	Prostitution	Wage diff.	Wage diff.
10	*Tobacco*	Prostitution	*Medical drugs*	*Medical drugs*	*Tobacco*	Prostitution
11	Gender equal.	Gender equal.	Prostitution	Gender equal.	*Medical drugs*	*Med. drugs*
12	Prostitution	*Gambling*	*Gambling*	Wage diff.	Gender equal.	Gender equal.
13	*Gambling*	Wage diff.	*Tobacco*	*Gambling*	Prostitution	*Tobacco*
14	*Medical drugs*	*Tobacco*	Gender equal.	*Tobacco*	*Gambling*	*Gambling*

than most of the available alternatives, except for addictions to 'hard' drugs (Norway, Sweden, and to some extent Finland), alcohol (Finland and Germany), and cannabis (Sweden). Notably, addictions to tobacco and gambling, and to some extent medical drugs, are ranked among the least severe societal problems in most countries. Indeed, the only 'non-addictive' problems that are ranked lower in severity than gambling are large wage differences (Norway), and gender inequality (Germany). Addiction to cannabis ranks relatively higher as a social problem among Swedes than among other nationals, whereas illegal use of medical drugs ranks relatively lower among Poles, and to some extent Finns, than among other respondents.

10.3.2 The perceived addictiveness of various substances and activities

Table 10.6 shows respondents' perceptions of the risk for persons who use certain substances or practice certain activities to become addicted. It should be noted here that the overall ratings are the means for all substances or activities, except cocaine use and Internet use, for which data are missing from some countries.

As shown, among the substances and activities for which there are data for all five countries, alcohol is overall seen as the least addictive and heroin as the most addictive. Notably, Swedes seem on average to perceive the riskiness of potentially addictive substances and activities as lower than respondents from other countries do, and Poles as higher than others do. In particular, Swedes rate the risk of getting addicted to alcohol, gambling, and smoking as relatively modest. On the other hand, Poles perceive the risk of getting addicted to cigarettes, cannabis, gambling, medical drugs, and alcohol to be significantly higher than respondents from other countries do. In sum, Poles seem more inclined than others, and Swedes less inclined than others, to emphasize the risk of becoming addicted to substances or gambling.

10.3.3 Perceived options of recovery

Thus far, the analyses indicate that there are clear differences between many of the studied countries concerning how the common citizen looks upon the 'social severity' of various addictions, as well as in the ways in which they rate the risk of becoming addicted to various forms of substance use or behaviours. As indicated by the following tables, these differences appear also when it comes to how people rate the probability of recovering from various addictions.

It is today well known that a large proportion—in many instances, the vast majority—of people who recover from various addictions do so without professional help and outside the traditional treatment system (e.g. Blomqvist & Cameron, 2002; Sobell & Klingemann, 2007; Blomqvist et al., 2007). However, the option of 'self-change' seems not to be very well acknowledged neither among lay judges, nor (as shown by e.g. Cunningham et al., 1998, and Samuelsson et al., 2013), among professionals in the field.

As indicated by Table 10.7, most respondents in the present study seem to agree that there is very little chance of recovering without professional help from an addiction to 'hard' drugs (i.e. heroin, cocaine, and amphetamines), whereas the options for untreated recovery from addictions to smoking or Internet use are seen as much better. As for between-country comparisons, Finns stand out as the most optimistic, rating the possibility for untreated

Table 10.6 Perceived risk of becoming addicted to various substances or activities (scale: 1–4; ' very small' (1) to 'very high' (4) risk)

Country	Poland	Norway	Germany	Finland	Sweden	All	p-value
Addiction to							
Heroin	3.46 (0.9)	3.68 (0.7)	3.61 (0.7)	3.64 (0.7)	3.41 (0.8)	3.56 (0.8)	< 0.001[a]
(Cocaine)	3.35 (0.9)	3.53 (0.8)	3.40 (0.7)	n a	3.33 (0.8)	3.40 (0.8)	< 0.001[b]
Amphetamines	3.36 (0.9)	3.47 (0.8)	2.95 (0.8)	3.41 (0.8)	3.19 (0.8)	3.27 (0.8)	< 0.001[c]
Cannabis	3.31 (0,9)	3.04 (0.9)	2.87 (0.9)	2.99 (0.9)	2.91 (0.9)	3.02 (0.9)	< 0.001[d]
Cigarettes	3.32 (0.8)	3.03 (0.8)	2.89 (0.8)	2.66 (1.0)	2.55 (0.9)	2.85 (0.9)	< 0.001[e]
Medical Drugs	3.00 (0.9)	2.55 (0.8)	2.60 (0.8)	2.47 (0.8)	2.37 (0.9)	2.60 (0.9)	< 0.001[f]
(Internet Use)	3.01 (0.9)	2.51 (0.9)	2.68 (0.9)	2.02 (1.0)	n a	2.58 (1.0)	< 0.001[g]
Gambling	3.09 (0.9)	2.49 (0.8)	2.68 (0.9)	2.16 (0.8)	2.12 (0.8)	2.51 (0.9)	< 0.001[h]
Alcohol	2.98 (0.9)	2.17 (0.6)	2.19 (0.9)	2.18 (0.8)	2.07 (0.8)	2.31 (0.9)	< 0.001[i]
Overall	*3.24 (0.6)*	*2.92 (0.5)*	*2.82 (0.6)*	*2.78 (0.6)*	*2.66 (0.6)*	*2.88 (0.7)*	*< 0.001*[j]

Scheffé post hoc tests: [a]N, F, G > P, S; [b]N > G, P, S; [c]N, F, P > S > G; [d]P > N, F > S, G; [e]P > N > G, F > S; [f]P > G > N > F, S; [g]P > G > N > F; [h]P > G > N > F, S; [i]P > G, F, N, G > S; [j]P > N > G, F > S.

Table 10.7 Perceived chances of untreated recovery from an addiction to various substances or activities (scale: 1–5; from 'none or very small' (1) to 'very big' (5))

Country	Poland	Norway	Germany	Finland	Sweden	All	p-value
Addiction to							
Cigarettes	2.89 (1.3)	3.65 (1.0)	2.77 (1.2)	3.57 (1.1)	3.82 (1.1)	3.34 (1.2)	$< 0.001^a$
(Internet Use)	2.72 (1.2)	3.38 (1.1)	2.60 (1.0)	3.62 (1.2)	n a	3.04 (1.3)	$< 0.001^b$
Gambling	2.23 (1.2)	2.82 (1.0)	2.10 (1.0)	3.42 (1.1)	3.02 (1.1)	2.69 (1.2)	$< 0.001^c$
Cannabis	2.09 (1.2)	2.64 (1.1)	2.26 (1.2)	2.58 (1.3)	2.58 (1.1)	2.43 (1.2)	$< 0.001^d$
Alcohol	2.11 (1.1)	2.70 (1.0)	1.85 (1.0)	2.88 (1.1)	2.64 (1.1)	2.42 (1.1)	$< 0.001^e$
Medical Drugs	2.18 (2.3)	2.37 (2.5)	1.94 (2.1)	2.68 (2.8)	2.36 (2.5)	2.32 (2.4)	$< 0.001^f$
Amphetamines	1.90 (1.1)	1.97 (0.9)	2.06 (1.0)	2.13 (1.3)	2.07 (1.1)	2.02 (1.1)	$< 0.001^g$
(Cocaine)	1.83 (1.1)	1.96 (0.9)	1.71 (1.0)	n a	1.92 (1.2)	1.86 (1.1)	$< 0.001^h$
Heroin	1.79 (1.1)	1.69 (0.9)	1.55 (1.0)	1.94 (1.3)	1.81 (1.2)	1.74 (1.1)	$< 0.001^i$
Overall	2.16 (0.9)	2.55 (0.7)	2.06 (0.8)	2.70 (0.8)	2.60 (0.8)	2.40 (0.8)	$< 0.001^j$

Scheffé post hoc tests: [a]S > N, F > P, G; [b]F > N > P, G; [c]F > S > N > P, G; [d]N, F, S > G, P; [e]F > N, S > P > G; [f]F > N, S > P > G; [g]F, S >G, N > P; [h]N, S > P, G; [i]F, S > P, N > G; [j]F, S > N > P, G.

recovery from addictions to heroin, medical drugs, gambling, and Internet use significantly higher than respondents from other countries. When it comes to recovery from addictions to alcohol cannabis, and heroin, Swedes stand out to be as optimistic as Finns, and when it comes to addiction to cigarettes, Swedes are the most optimistic. Also, concerning cocaine addiction, where there are no data from Finland, Swedes, together with Norwegians, show the strongest trust in 'self-change'. Considering all addictions, Finns and Swedes seem more inclined than others, and Poles and Germans less inclined than others to believe in the option of untreated recovery.

Whereas the notion of 'self-change' is largely met with doubt, the trust in professional treatment of addictive problems is rather strong, almost independent of type of addiction. As indicated by Table 10.8, there are also relatively small differences between the five countries in this respect. With exception for the case of heroin addiction, Norwegians seem, rather generally to have a somewhat higher confidence in the benefits of addiction treatment than respondents from other countries. Thus they rate the probability of recovering with the help of professional treatment as significantly higher than others do when it comes to addictions to cigarettes, gambling, and Internet use.

10.3.4 **Who is held responsible?**

Table 10.9 illustrates how respondents attribute the responsibility for getting addicted to various substances or activities. As shown, lay people seem prone to blame the individual user for addictions to the Internet, gambling, and cigarettes, whereas addiction to medical drugs and alcohol is more often seen as at least partly due to circumstances. Blaming the individual more strongly for substance addictions than for behavioural addictions may indicate that the former are to a larger degree seen as 'diseases'.

Between-country differences are rather small, apart from the interesting fact that Finns seem overall to be significantly more inclined, and Swedes significantly less inclined than others, to blame the individual for acquiring an addiction. This points to rather different sentiments between two neighbouring welfare countries concerning the moral attitudes towards substance use problems. It is also worth noting that 'untreated' and 'treated' recovery do not seem to be perceived as opposite alternatives, but rather that the main differences between addictions and countries seem to be about overall change optimism or pessimism (see tables 10.7 and 10.8).

Finally, Table 10.10 illustrates respondents' perceptions of the extent to which the individual addict should be held responsible for solving an addiction problem. As can be seen, most respondents seem to have a rather 'moral' perception (in contrast to a 'disease' view) of how to handle addiction problems, insofar as they rather generally attribute the main responsibility for solving the problem

Table 10.8 Perceived chances of treated recovery from an addiction to various substances or activities (scale: 1–5; from 'none or very small' (1) to 'very big' (5))

Country	Poland	Norway	Germany	Finland	Sweden	All	p-value
Addiction to							
Alcohol	3.82 (1.)	4.05 (0,8)	3.68 (0.9)	3.92 (0.9)	3.98 (0.9)	3.89 (0.9)	< 0.001[a]
Cigarettes	3.62 (1.1)	4.17 (0.9)	3.66 (1.0)	3.61 (1.1)	3.98 (1.1)	3.82 (1.1)	< 0.001[b]
Cannabis	3.69 (1.1)	3.91 (0.9)	3.60 (1.0)	3.77 (1.1)	3.83 (1.0)	3.76 (1.0)	< 0.001[c]
Medical Drugs	3.71 (1.0)	3.91 (0.8)	3.58 (1.0)	3.61 (0.9)	3.84 (1.0)	3.74 (1.0)	< 0.001[d]
Gambling	3.57 (1.1)	4.05 (0.8)	3.52 (1.0)	3.53 (1.1)	3.90 (0.9)	3.74 (1.0)	< 0.001[e]
(Internet Use)	3.59 (1.1)	3.96 (1.0)	3.49 (1.1)	3.55 (1.3)	n a	3.65 (1.1)	< 0.001[f]
Amphetamine	3.68 (1.1)	3.63 (1,0)	3.57 (1.0)	3.62 (1.0)	3.67 (1.0)	3.64 (1.0)	n s
(Cocaine)	3.62 (1.1)	3.58 (1.0)	3.26 (1.1)	n a	3.57 (1.1)	3.51 (1.1)	< 0.001[g]
Heroin	3.63 (1.2)	3.38 (1.1)	3.17 (1.2)	3.48 (1.2)	3.52 (1.2)	3.43 (1.2)	< 0.001[h]
Overall	*3.69 (0.9)*	*3.89 (0.7)*	*3.55 (0.8)*	*3.67 (0.8)*	*3.52 (1.2)*	*3.73 (0.8)*	*< 0.001[i]*

Scheffé post hoc tests: [a]N, S > D > F, G; [b]N > S > G, P, F; [c]N, S, F > P, G; [d]N, S > D > F, G; [e]N > S > F, P, G; [f]N > P, F, G; [g]P, N, S > G, P, F; [h]P > S, F, N > G; [i]N, S > P, F > G.

Table 10.9 Perceived reasons/responsibility for acquiring an addiction (1 = 'mainly the person's fault'; 4 = 'mainly due to circumstances')

Country	Poland	Norway	Germany	Finland	Sweden	All	p-value
Addiction to							
Medical drugs	2.14 (1.0)	2.17 (0.9)	2.06 (0.9)	1.88 (0.9)	2.43 (0.9)	2.15 (0.9)	< 0.001[a]
'Hard' drugs	*n a*	*n a*	*n a*	*2.06 (1.0)*	*n a*	*n a*	*n a*
Heroin	*1.78 (1.1)*	*2.06 (1.0)*	*2.08 (1.0)*	*n a*	*2.13 (0.9)*	*2.02 (1.0)*	*< 0.001[b]*
Alcohol	1.99 (1.0)	1.88 (0.7)	2.05 (0.9)	1.97 (0.8)	2.13 (0.8)	2.01 (0.8)	< 0.001[c]
Cannabis	1.90 (1.0)	1.97 (0.9)	2.05 (0.9)	2.02 (1.0)	2.09 (0.8)	2.01 (0.9)	< 0.001[d]
Cocaine	*1.81 (1.0)*	*2.03 (1.0)*	*1.99 (1.0)*	*n a*	*2.11 (1.0)*	*1.99 (0.9)*	*< 0.001[e]*
Amphetamine	*1.81 (1.0)*	*2.00 (0.9)*	*2.00 (0.9)*	*n a*	*2.11 (0.9)*	*1.98 (0.9)*	*< 0.001[f]*
Cigarettes	1.73 (0.9))	1.75 (0.8)	1.93 (0.9)	1.79 (0.9)	1.73 (0.8)	1.79 (0.8)	< 0.001[g]
Gambling	1.73 (0.9)	1.67 (0.7)	1.77 (0.8)	1.55 (0.7)	1.75 (0.8)	1.70 (0.8)	< 0.001[h]
Internet Use	1.62 (0.8)	1.66 (0.8)	1.80 (0.8)	1.52 (0.8)	n a	1.66 (0.8)	< 0.001[i]
Overall	*1.89 (0.6)*	*1.88 (0.5)*	*1.96 (0.6)*	*1.83 (0.6)*	*2.03 (0.6)*	*1.93 (0.6)*	*< 0.001[j]*

Scheffé post hoc tests: [a]S > N, P, G > F; [b]S > N, G > P; [c]S > G, P, F > N; [d]S, G, F > N, P; [e f g]G > F, N, P, S; [h]G, S, P, N > F; [i]G > F, N, P, S; [j]S > G, P, N > F.

Table 10.10 Perceived responsibility for solving an addiction problem (1 = 'mainly the person's responsibility'; 2 = 'mainly society's responsibility')

Country	**Poland**	**Norway**	**Germany**	**Finland**	**Sweden**	**All**	**p-value**
Addiction to							
'Hard' drugs	*n a*	*n a*	*n a*	*2.14 (0.9)*	*n a*	*n a*	*n a*
Medical Drugs	1.72 (0.8)	2.26 (0.9)	2.02 (0.9)	1.98 (0.8)	2.23 (0,8)	2.05 (1.0)	< 0.001[a]
Heroin	*1.76 (0.9)*	*2.06 (0.9)*	*2.08 (1.0)*	*n a*	*2.16 (0.8)*	*2.02 (0.9)*	*< 0.001[b]*
Cocaine	1.73 (0.9)	1.98 (0.9)	1.99 (1.0)	n a	2.14 (0.8)	1.97 (0.9)	< 0.001[c]
Cannabis	1.74 (0.9)	1.77 (0.8)	1.89 (0.9)	2.00 (0.8)	1.99 (0.7)	1.87 (0.8)	< 0.001[d]
Alcohol	1.82 (0,9)	1.73 (0,7)	1.97 (0.9)	1.87 (1.6)	1.91 (0.6)	1.86 (0.8)	< 0.001[e]
Gambling	1.59 (0.8)	1.83 (0.8)	1.95 (1.0)	1.66 (0.7)	1.78 (0.7)	1.77 (0.8)	< 0.001[f]
Internet Use	1.60 (0.8)	1.51 (0.7)	1.87 (1.0)	1.49 (0.7)	n a	1.62 (0.8)	< 0.001[g]
Cigarettes	1.55 (0.8)	1.50 (0.7)	1.79 (0.9)	1.46 (0.7)	1.40 (0.6)	1.54 (0.7)	< 0.001[h]
Overall	*1.69 (0.7)*	*1.81 (0.7)*	*1.93 (0.7)*	*1.78 (0.6)*	*1.86 (0.5)*	*1.82 (0.6)*	*< 0.001[i]*

Scheffé post hoc tests: [a]S, G > F, N > P; [b]G, N > P; [c]G, N > P; [d]F, S, G > N, P; [e]G, S, F > P, N; [f]G > N, S > F, P; [g]N > G, P; [h]G > N, P > F; [i]G > F, N, P, S.

to the individual addict rather than to society. This 'moral' view seems to be strongest as concerns smoking and Internet use, and least strong as concerns heroin use and illegal use of prescribed medical drugs. In the latter case this may reflect a tendency to see the medical system as partly responsible for creating the problem. Regards between-country differences, Poles and Finns seem to endorse a somewhat more 'moral' view than Germans and Swedes.

Interestingly, and in some contrast to what has often reported to be the case in the USA, these European respondents seem rather reluctant to attribute the responsibility for, e.g. smoking and gambling problems to others than the individual smoker or gambler, such as e.g., the tobacco or gambling companies. In contrast, people who are addicted to alcohol and illegal drugs, seem to a much larger degree to be regarded as 'victims'.

10.4 **Discussion**

10.4.1 **Limitations**

The study, the main results of which have been presented in this chapter, is fraught with certain limitations. First, there is some uncertainty around to what extent the five national samples are comparable with regard to their representativeness of the respective populations. The Swedish, Finnish, and Norwegian samples are recruited randomly from census population data. In addition, data are weighted, using gender and age, as well as education (Sweden and Norway) and income, marital status, and country of origin (Sweden) as calibration variables. Although this should control for the most common type of attrition bias, it has probably not been able to prevent consumers of various substances from being underrepresented among the respondents. However, a previous analysis of the Swedish data, with and without weighting, yielded largely similar results (Blomqvist, 2009). As for data from Germany and Poland, where random digit dialling was used, potential bias is harder to control. However, these data have been weighted to guarantee that the samples include the same proportions as the respective populations with respect to gender and age distribution. All in all, there is little reason to believe that the differing sampling procedures have jeopardized the comparability of the national samples in a serious way.

Another limitation is that the different response modes (postal survey, telephone interview, and web panel), and consequential differences with regard to how the questions were phrased, may have induced differences in how certain questions were interpreted by respondents in different countries. This type of potential influence is hard to evaluate, but the most probable impact is that the Polish and German data may include somewhat fewer misinterpreted questions, because the telephone mode to a greater extent enables clarification of potentially misunderstood questions. It must also be acknowledged that the number of statistical tests conveys a risk of mass significances, and that it needs to be further analyzed which differences are significant also in a policy and practice context. Another potential source of bias that may have raised respondents' concerns over substance use problems in comparison with other social problems is the fact that the focus in the questionnaires clearly was on addictive problems. Finally, it should be observed that policies and attitudes may to some extent have changed during the six-year period between the first data collection in 2007 (Sweden) and the last ones in 2013 (Germany and Poland).

10.4.2 **Main conclusions**

Acknowledging the limitations, a summary description of the results presented in this report would read as follows.

It is rather obvious from the analyses that 'addiction' is not seen as a unitary phenomenon by lay people in any of the five countries. Rather, there are relatively large differences, in all of the countries, between the judgements of most of the investigated addictions, in the majority of the explored dimensions. In particular, there seem to be large differences in the perception of the severity to society of different addictions, where addictions to 'hard' drugs (heroin, amphetamines, and cocaine) are, with a few exceptions, seen as by far the most dangerous problems to society, and behavioural addictions, such as addictions to gambling and Internet use, generally come out as much less severe. Largely the same differences, although less pronounced, appear concerning the perceived risk of becoming addicted to various substances or activities. In comparable aspects these perceptions are also to a large extent at odds with the results of recent attempts to rank the overall harms (for society and the user) of the use of various mind-altering substances, pointing to alcohol as by far the most detrimental substance (Nutt et al., 2010).

When it comes to the perceived chances for recovery, the confidence in treatment is relatively high for all addictions, whereas the probability of 'self-change' from addictions to 'hard' drugs, and to some extent medical drugs and alcohol, are generally rated as very or fairly small. On the other hand, the options of recovering from addictions to cigarettes or Internet use without treatment are generally rated as fairly high. However, there seems to be a main divide between different addictions as concerns overall 'change optimism' (with and without treatment) and 'change pessimism'. Finally, most respondents seem to have a rather 'moral' view on addiction problems, holding the individual, rather than other circumstances responsible, both for acquiring and solving an addiction problem. The main exceptions here seem to be addictions to medical drugs, 'hard' narcotic drugs, and alcohol, where the individual is more often seen as a victim.

In addition, the results imply that the dominant perceptions of addictions vary between the five countries. Thus, for example, Swedes seem overall to be more concerned, and Germans and Finns less concerned, than others over addiction as a severe societal problem. More specifically, Swedes, Norwegians, and Germans rate addiction to 'hard' narcotic drugs as a more dangerous societal problem than other addictions, whereas Poles and Finns reserve this place for addiction to alcohol. When compared with other societal problems, addictions to 'hard' drugs and alcohol are generally judged to be among the most severe, next to violent crimes (Norway and Sweden) and/or poverty (Poland and Finland). At the same time, addictions to gambling, tobacco, medical drugs, and Internet use, are ranked as less severe than most other societal problems. As for the 'addictiveness' of various substance use habits and other activities, Poles seem overall to be more concerned, and Swedes less concerned than people in the other countries.

When it comes to the perceived chances of solving an addiction problem, Norwegians seem overall to have greater trust, and Swedes and Germans lower trust, than respondents from other countries in professional treatment, whereas Finns and Swedes are overall more optimistic than others concerning the possibility of 'self-change'. Interestingly, Finns, who see addiction to alcohol as the addiction problem that is most dangerous to society, also seem to have a stronger belief than respondents from other countries that people are able to solve such problems without professional help. In line with this, Finns (and to some extent Poles) also seem to take a more 'moral' view than others towards addiction (not least to alcohol), attributing the responsibility for acquiring and solving these problems largely to the individual addict, whereas Germans and Swedes seem more inclined to blame other circumstances for the onset of addiction problems, and/or to underline society's responsibility for solving them.

Overall, these findings are worthy of further consideration, exploration, and discussion in the face of some prevailing tendencies in the addiction field at large. One of these is the strong inclination, in both national and international discussions, to account for addiction as a global problem—and to issue policies and guidelines predominantly on the global level. Since addiction problems might be seen as typically 'interactive' (Hacking, 1999)—that is, the dominant definitions of addiction tend to influence the behaviour of those defined—and since popular support has recurrently been shown to be a necessary condition for effective implementation of national policies, this may not be an optimal strategy under present circumstances.

Another, potentially premature tendency—which the present data may place under some doubt—is the inclination to lump various 'addictive' problems together, in policy documents as well as theoretical discussions, under one common heading (e.g. 'progressive brain disease'; see Heim et al., 2014; Rehm et al., 2013), with an allegedly common explanatory basis. Not least from what has been called a 'contextual constructionist perspective' (Best, 1995), a fruitful understanding and handling of addiction problems must take into account a number of interacting factors, including the social and historical context where these problems manifest themselves and are defined and dealt with. Some examples of salient dimensions that might need to be included in such a deeper understanding have been discussed by Sulkunen (2013) under the heading 'geographies of addiction'.

10.5 Acknowledgements

Jan Blomqvist and Kirsimarja Raitasalo are main authors of this chapter. Hans Olav Melberg, Dirk Schreckenberg, Christine Peschel, Justyna Klingemann, and Anja Koski-Jännes have been responsible for the analysis of their country's data sets.

Notes

1 Alcohol; cannabis; other ('hard') narcotic drugs: heroin, amphetamines, cocaine; cigarettes; (illegally used) medical drugs; gambling; and Internet use as societal problems.

2 Addiction and Lifestyles in Contemporary Europe—Reframing Addictions Project.

References

Alexander, B. (2008). The globalization of addiction: a study in poverty of the spirit. Oxford: Oxford University Press.

Best, J. (1995). Constructionism in context. In J. Best (Ed.), Images of issues: typifying contemporary social problems. New York: Aldine DeGruyter. 335–354.

Blomqvist J. (2009). What is the worst thing you could get hooked on? Popular images of addiction problems in contemporary Sweden. *Nordic Studies on Alcohol and Drugs*, **26**(4), 373–398.

Blomqvist, J. (2002). Recovery with and without treatment: a comparison of resolutions of alcohol and drug problems. *Addiction Research and Theory*, **10**(2), 119–168.

Blomqvist, J. (2004). Sweden's 'war on drugs' in the light of addicts' own experiences. In P. Rosenqvist et al., (Eds.), Addiction and life course. Publication **44**. Helsinki: NAD. 139–171.

Blomqvist, J. et al. (2007) Att förbättra sina dryckesvanor: om olika mönster för förändring och vad vården betyder. Stockholms universitet, SoRAD: Rapport no 42.

Blomqvist, J. (2012). Perceptions of addiction and recovery in Sweden: the influence of respondent characteristics. *Addiction Research and Theory*, **20**(53), 435–466.

Blomqvist, J. and Cameron, D. (2002) Editorial: Moving away from addiction: forces, processes, and contexts. Addiction Research and Theory, **10**(2), 115–118.

Blomqvist, J., Koski-Jännes, A., & Cunningham, J. (2014). How should substance use problems be handled? Popular views in Sweden, Finland, and Canada. *Drugs and Alcohol Today*, **14**(1), 19–30.

Cunningham, J., Blomqvist, J., Koski-Jännes, A., & Raitasalo, K. (2012). Societal images of cannabis use: comparing three countries. *Harm Reduction Journal*, **9**(21),

Cunningham, J.A., Sobell, L.C., & Sobell, M.B. (1998). Awareness of self-change as a pathway to recovery for alcohol abusers: results from five different groups. *Addictive Behaviors*, **23**, 399–404.

Cunningham, J.A. (2009). Societal images of addiction—first results from a Canadian representative survey. Paper presented at the 35th Annual Alcohol Epidemiology Symposium of the Kettil Bruun Society, Copenhagen, 1–5 June 2009.

Hacking, I. (1999). The social construction of what? London: Harvard University Press.

Heim, D. et al. (2014). Addiction: not just brain malfunction. *Nature*, **507**(40), (06 March 2014) doi:10.1038/507040e.

Holma, K., Koski-Jännes, A., Raitasalo, K., Blomqvist, J., Pervova, I., & Cunningham, J. (2009). Perceptions of addictions as societal problems in Canada, Sweden, Finland and Russia, *European Addiction Research*, **17**(2), 106–112.

Klingemann, H. (1992). Coping and maintenance strategies of spontaneous remitters from problem use of alcohol and heroin in Switzerland. *International Journal of the Addictions*, **27**, 1359–1388.

Koski-Jännes, A., Hirschovits-Gerz, T., Pennonen, M., & Nyyssönen, M. (2012). Population, professional and clients' views on dangerousness of various addictions on individual and society. *Nordic Studies on Alcohol and Drugs*, **29**(2), 139–154.

Moscovici, S. (1981). On social representations. In J.P. Forgas (Ed.), Social cognition. London: Academic Press. 181–209.

Moscovici, S. (1988). Notes towards a description of social representations. *European Journal of Social Psychology*, **18**(3), 211–250.

Nutt, D.J., King, L.A., & Philips, L.D. (2010). Drug harms in the UK: a multicriteria decision analysis. *The Lancet*, **9752**, 1558–1565.

Rehm, J. et al. (2013). Defining substance use disorders: do we really need more than heavy use? *Alcohol and Alcoholism*, **48**(6), 633–640.

Room, R. (1978). Governing images of alcohol and drug problems [doctoral dissertation]. University of California, Berkeley.

Samuelsson, E. Blomqvist, J., & Christophs, I. (2013). Addiction and recovery—conceptions among professionals in the Swedish treatment system. *Nordic Studies on Alcohol and Drugs*, **26**(4), 373–938.

Sobell, L.C. and Klingemann, Harald (2007) Promoting Self-Change from Addictive Behaviors. Practical Implications for Policy, Prevention, and Treatment. Springer.

Sulkunen, P. (2013). Geographies of addiction. *Nordic Studies on Alcohol and Drugs*, **30**(7–12).

Index

Page numbers in italics indicate Figures; those in bold type indicate Tables.

D

E

The manufacturer's authorised representative in the EU for product safety is Oxford University Press España S.A. of El Parque Empresarial San Fernando de Henares, Avenida de Castilla, 2 - 28830 Madrid (www.oup.es/en or product.safety@oup.com). OUP España S.A. also acts as importer into Spain of products made by the manufacturer.
Printed and bound by CPI Group (UK) Ltd, Croydon, CR0 4YY
14/09/2026
02216287-0009